Social Indicators Research Series

Volume 63

This series aims to provide a public forum for single treatises and collections of papers on social indicators research that are too long to be published in our journal *Social Indicators Research*. Like the journal, the book series deals with statistical assessments of the quality of life from a broad perspective. It welcomes research on a wide variety of substantive areas, including health, crime, housing, education, family life, leisure activities, transportation, mobility, economics, work, religion and environmental issues. These areas of research will focus on the impact of key issues such as health on the overall quality of life and vice versa. An international review board, consisting of Ruut Veenhoven, Joachim Vogel, Ed Diener, Torbjorn Moum and Wolfgang Glatzer, will ensure the high quality of the series as a whole.

More information about this series at http://www.springer.com/series/6548

Bernhard Schmitz

Art-of-Living

A Concept to Enhance Happiness

Springer

Bernhard Schmitz
Institute for Psychology
Darmstadt University of Technology
Darmstadt
Germany

ISSN 1387-6570 ISSN 2215-0099 (electronic)
Social Indicators Research Series
ISBN 978-3-319-45323-1 ISBN 978-3-319-45324-8 (eBook)
DOI 10.1007/978-3-319-45324-8

Library of Congress Control Number: 2016949609

Printed on acid-free paper

This Springer imprint is published by Springer Nature
The registered company is Springer International Publishing AG
The registered company address is: Gewerbestrasse 11, 6330 Cham, Switzerland

Foreword

On the growing importance of 'art-of living'

This book is about how to live a good life, a satisfying life in particular. The art of living is a topic that has interested man since ancient times and that has figured prominently in classic Greek philosophy. Today the issue is even more pertinent.

Happiness depends on life-ability

For a long time happiness was seen as a matter of luck, as is illustrated by the history of the word, 'happiness,' which comes from 'happening.' Today we see happiness as a result of our own actions. One reason for this change of view is that social conditions now allow us more control over our lives and another is that recent happiness research has allowed us to estimate better how much control we have.

Happiness research has shown that most people live happy lives in contemporary Western nations; average happiness is around 7, 5 on a scale of 0–10[1], and it has increased slightly over the last 50 years. The main reason is that that living conditions are pretty good in modern Western nations. Yet not everybody is equally happy in Western nations; for instance, in Germany some 36 % of the population is very happy, scoring 9 or 10 on the happiness scale, while 15 % are unhappy and rate their happiness at 5 or less. Though these differences have become a bit smaller over time, they are still considerable, as is apparent from an average standard deviation of 2 for the German population.[2]

Why is there such a difference in happiness among people living in the same nation? One answer is that living conditions differ within countries; some citizens being better situated than their compatriots, e.g., have a higher income or a more

[1]http://worlddatabaseofhappiness.eur.nl/hap_nat/desc_na_genpublic.php?cntry=636&region=2748.

[2]http://worlddatabaseofhappiness.eur.nl/common/desc_study.php?studyid=10921.

supportive family. Likewise some people are just luckier than fellow citizens, e.g., win a lottery or happen to work in a booming industry. Yet these differences in living conditions within countries explain at best about 25 % of the differences in happiness in the population. This means that about 75 % of the differences in happiness lies in what people make of their situation. We also know that about 35 % of the differences in happiness lies in genetic factors, which we cannot change. This leaves us with the suggestion that about 40 % of the differences lies in things that are within our control.[3]

Happiness is becoming more dependent on life-ability

This share of 40 % is not a fixed number; it was probably lower in the past and is likely to get bigger in the future. One reason is that the degree to which we are in control of our happiness depends on our life situation. The better the external living conditions in a society, the higher the average happiness will be, but the more the remaining differences in happiness across citizens will depend on their life ability. In the best possible situation, say in heaven, there will still be differences in happiness, say between people scoring 9 or 10. These differences will be near to 100 % due to variation in life ability. Since living conditions have improved over time, happiness has become more dependent on life ability and if living conditions will improve further in the future, happiness will become even more dependent on our talent for living.

A related reason for the growing importance of life ability is that we have more choice than ever before: We live in a 'multiple-choice-society' and can decide on many things that were preset for earlier generations, such as the type of work we do, whom we marry, and whether or not we have children. This greater freedom of choice is one of the reasons why most people are happy, but it also requires skills to choose. It is easier to follow custom.

We value happiness more

Happiness is a universal value; almost all humans prefer a satisfying life over a miserable life. Yet happiness is not valued equally at all times and in all places. Happiness ranks relatively high in the value hierarchy of contemporary Western nations, among other things because living a happy life is very possible in the conditions of modern society.[4]

All these have created a growing demand for information on how to live a happy life and this information demand is increasingly served by scientific research. Two new strands of happiness research have developed recently, 'happiness economics'

[3]Veenhoven, R. (2015) Social conditions for human happiness: a review of research. International Journal of Psychology, 50(3), 379–391, Section 5.3.

[4]Veenhoven, R. (2015) Happiness: History of the concept, in: James Wright (Ed.) International Encyclopedia of Social and Behavioural Sciences, 2nd edition Vol. 10, 521–525.

and 'positive psychology.' This book is part of the latter strand. It describes the current state of the art and presents interesting new findings. It will not be the last book on the 'art-of-living' but it makes an important contribution to our growing knowledge on this subject.

Ruut Veenhoven
Emeritus professor of social conditions
for human happiness
Erasmus University Rotterdam
The Netherlands

Acknowledgements

I am grateful for the assistance of so many people who supported me finishing this book. Therefore, I want to say thank you to each of you. At first, I want to show my gratitude to Anna Schmid who supported me developing an art-of-living questionnaire. At second, I am grateful for the organizational and content work of my research assistants Angelika Kern, Bettina Schumacher, Josephine Berger and Jessica Lang.

Special thanks to Janina Linten who was very engaged with the organization of some chapters of a previous version of the book and who supported the collaboration of the research group by her extraordinary social competence. Also I would like to thank all of the student assistants for working on this book and also for their graduation works who helped me to study art-of-living from so many different perspectives: Agnieszka Daniel, Alexander Stahlmann, Alice Lautz, Alina Stöver, Anna Petryszyn, Anne Traulsen, Boyan Ventsislavov Dimov, Carolin Rupp, Corinna Gräfe, Gesche Janzarik, Jana Demel, Julia Ankenbrand, Katharina Treichel, Magdalena Krankenhagen, André Markus, Monica Da Silva-Bettner, Nafiseh Küffner, Nicole Klimek, Remigija Rudaityte-Pusch, Sarah Haardt, Victoria Misch, Angelici Tsiouris, Luisa Margarian, Charlotte Kliem, Andre Markus, Max Lohner, Leah Strubelt, Linnea Landeberg, Kira Ahrens, Alina Wuttke, Thomas Proksch, Jennifer Bisch, Darya Yatsevich, Laura Hosemann and Ute Leischer were very helpful in the final production phase.

Contents

Ways for Living a Good Life

What defines a good life? What is the best sort of a person to be? These questions arouse since ancient times (Michalos 2015). This book series deals with exactly these questions: How can one achieve happiness and well-being and what determines the quality of life? According to Michalos, answers to early philosophers imply that a good life, on the one hand, should include wealth and physical attractiveness, and, on the other hand, a good life means living in peace and living in harmony with the conditions of the world and is based on an immortal soul.

Because of the importance of these questions, one goal of this book is to analyze ways how people can strive for a good life.

This question cannot be answered easily. Firstly, we give an overview of already-existing important concepts in psychology which may be related to living a good life. Secondly, we introduce our own approach: the concept of art-of-living as one way to achieve happiness.

The main reason for the necessity to elaborate this concept is related to the ideas of Veenhoven (2003a, b), who has edited a special issue in the Journal of Happiness Studies on the topic leading a good life. He points out that it is essential to discriminate between the outcomes of leading a good life and ways to achieve it. For example, if someone is exercising, e.g., runs long distances, this could eventually lead to (at least momentary) happiness. In this case, exercising would be the means and momentarily happiness the result.

Why is Veenhoven's discrimination between means and ends so important? Because some means can be learned and taught, whereas it could be very difficult to learn or teach the result, how to be happy, directly. Therefore, it is important to have a group of variables which can be learned and hence be trained and which may lead to happiness.

This book is conceptualized the following way: This introductory part points out important advantages why to study art-of-living. The following theoretical part illustrates our idea of the concept of art-of-living in greater detail. Then we present empirical studies evaluating a questionnaire to measure art-of-living, especially demonstrating its reliability and validity for a large group of concepts and different methods. In the final part, we present empirical studies showing that art-of-living and therefore, happiness can be enhanced and by which means that can be accomplished. We performed intervention studies for different groups, for students at school, at the university, and for working people, and we describe in detail the contents of our interventions. In a final chapter, we describe the results of interviews with people which were nominated from a sample as examples for artists-of-living. Then we search for the art-of-living in the arts, especially in autobiographies of famous people and we present an outlook for further research.

References

Michalos, A. C. (2015). *Ancient views on the quality of life.* Springer International Publishing.
Veenhoven, R. (2003a). Arts-of-living. *Journal of Happiness Studies,* (4), 373–384.
Veenhoven, R. (2003b). Notions of art-of-living. *Journal of Happiness Studies, 4*(4), 345–349.

Chapter 1
Introduction: Advantages of Using the Concept Art-of-Living

1.1 Introduction

In this introductory chapter, we firstly refer to Veenhoven's (2003a, b) important discrimination between leading a good life and its results, which could be happiness. Secondly, because we are interested in ways for leading a good life, we look at criteria which define what a good life is. Thirdly, as we are not the first ones who search ways for leading a good life, we consider some psychological concepts which have dealt in the literature with the ways of performing a good life. Then we discuss a group of more fine-grained and behavior-oriented strategies helpful for leading a good life. Finally, we summarize our considerations and derive aspects which could be seen as a foundation for our own integrative approach: the art-of-living. To elaborate the concept of art-of-living we took into consideration Veenhoven's (2003a, b) classification and refer to the philosophical background of art-of-living.

1.1.1 Background: Veenhoven's Discrimination for Ways to Lead a Good Life and its Results

Before we can introduce our approach for leading a good life we present Veenhoven's important discrimination between ways to achieve a good life and their results, which could at best be happiness. Veenhoven (2003a, b) gives an introduction in the special issue of the Journal of happiness studies, see also Veenhoven (2014).

For various reasons, Veenhoven (2003b, 2013) provides a basis for our concept of leading a good life, see Table 1.1. Firstly, the distinction he makes between life chances and life results is essential for our concept. Secondly, he discriminates between inner and outer qualities of life (Veenhoven 2003a). Outer qualities are

B. Schmitz, *Art-of-Living*, Social Indicators Research Series 63,
DOI 10.1007/978-3-319-45324-8_1

Table 1.1 Veenhoven's (2003b, 2013, p. 199) classification of ways for leading a good life

	Outer qualities	Inner qualities
Life chances	Livability of the environment	Life-ability of the person, Art-of-living[a]
Life results	Utility of life	Appreciation of life

Note: [a]Not contained in the original table. Added by the author

environmental factors that have an influence on the quality of life whereas inner qualities depend on the individual. For our model it is noteworthy that Veenhoven conceptualizes life-abilities in the upper right quadrant. That means life-ability is classified as inner qualities as well as life chances. This table will be referred to later. Based on Veenhoven's classification we argue that it is necessary to distinguish between ways to achieve a good life and results of such an attempt. Veenhoven regards leading a good life as a mental skill and underlines that this is perceived as a positive concept and is similar to the construct of positive mental health. People can influence their happiness, and he points out that it "may be a practical venue for intervention" (Veenhoven 2003a, p. 349) which can be learnt at least partially. Summarizing his concept of leading a good life he emphasizes (a) that *there is not only one way to a good life* and (b) *ways of leading a good life can be viewed as skills* and (c) that *the difference between ways and results of leading a good life is very important.*

One could also refer to the factors considered in Lyubomirsky's (2008) model of influences on happiness, which argues that 50 % of happiness are determined by genes which cannot be influenced by the individual (forming the fix-point), 10 % are environmental factors and further 40 % are conscious behavior, which can be influenced by the individual. Ways of leading a good life would therefore be classified in the 40 % behavioral factor.

1.2 Criteria for Happiness as Indirect Advice for Ways to Achieve Happiness

It seems to be clear, that ways of leading a good life are determined by the kind of good life which is sought for. Because there are different kinds of a good life, we discuss these kinds as criteria for happiness. One could suppose the criteria give information about what could be done to achieve happiness. For example, one might speculate that to achieve hedonic happiness (see below) it could be helpful to perform joyful activities like going to parties and listen to nice music, where as to achieve eudaimonia, it would be helpful to reflect one's life and to find meaning in life. Therefore, it is also important how people conceive happiness and, from a more scientific angle, how happiness is measured. Attempting to measure latent variables like, in this case, happiness, one can use objective or subjective measures. It seems likely that objective measures of happiness could be income and occupation, but researchers have found that various objective life measures (like income, age, occupation) were only weakly related to people's judgment of their lives, which leads to the necessity for subjective measures.

1.2.1 Subjective Well-Being (SWB)

Diener and Lucas (1999) define *Subjective well-being* (SWB) as life satisfaction, the absence of negative affect and the presence of positive affect, and his three component structure has been widely used in research. SWB refers to people's evaluation of their lives, containing affective and cognitive aspects, and is therefore seen as construct that represents everyday terms of happiness. It is not only related to short term pleasures but takes into consideration a broader picture of happiness (Diener 1984).

When trying to measure satisfaction with one's life, researchers often use a single item: "How satisfied are you with your life as a whole?" (Andrew and Withey 1976). A more refined instrument that is commonly used is the Satisfaction with life scale (SWLS) (Diener et al. 1985), consisting of five items. This scale has been widely applied and shows good reliability (alpha = .85).

1.2.2 Psychological Well-Being (PBW)

Ryff (1989) has criticized the concept of subjective well-being, mainly because of its missing theoretical foundation and because it therefore neglects important aspects of psychological functioning. Based on theories of Maslow (1968), Rogers (1961), Jung (1933) and Erikson (1959), she developed the concept of *psychological well-being* (PWB) which is much more differentiated and integrates concepts of psychological functioning from various theoretical backgrounds into an overall construct. Two important criteria of positive functioning are: holding positive attitudes towards oneself (self-acceptance) and having warm, and trusting interpersonal relations (positive relations with others). According to Ryff there is considerable agreement in the literature on other important criteria such as self-determination, independence and regulation of behavior from within (autonomy). Another characteristic of mental health is the individual's ability to choose or create environments suitable to its conditions (environmental mastery). Positive functioning also includes beliefs that give one the feeling that there is purpose and meaning in life (purpose in life). Ryff argues that it is a kind of psychological functioning if one tries to continue to develop one's potential and to grow (personal growth).

Therefore, PWB summarizes the following concepts of positive functioning: self-growth, self-acceptance, environment, relationships, meaning and autonomy. Clearly this concept of psychological well-being gives more information what could be done to achieve well-being. For example, to achieve relationship well-being one could improve one's relationships or to achieve self-growth, one can live in correspondence to one's needs and goals. Ryff's concept and instrument of PWB have been widely applied (cf. Baumgardner and Crothers 2010; Ryff and Singer 1996; Keyes et al. 2002).

1.2.3 Eudaimonia and Hedonia

The concept of *eudaimonic well-being* was introduced by Waterman (1990) and is based on the ideas of Aristotle, who uses the term "daimon" with the meaning of "the true self". According to Aristotle, a good life means living in accordance with your inner daimon and true happiness can be achieved from the realization of inner potentials, in other words, happiness derives from self-realization. As a result, one should live in line with one's needs, talents and values. Waterman argues that eudaimonic happiness results from personal expressiveness, for if people are fully engaged in activities and show their sense of what they are that will result in an experience of fulfillment and meaningfulness.

Huta and Waterman (2014) provide a thorough distinction between eudaimonia and hedonia: Following these authors eudaimonia is related to growth, meaning, authenticity and excellence whereas hedonia is characterized by pleasure, enjoyment, comfort and absence of distress. Both concepts can be dated back to philosophers dealing with the question about the nature of a good life or whether a life is well-lived. In hedonic philosophies the focus is on the above mentioned concepts pleasure, enjoyment, and absence of distress whereas in eudaimonic philosophies the focus is on activities reflecting virtue, excellence, the best within us, and the full development of our potentials. Although hedonic and eudaimonic happiness can theoretically and practically be discriminated the constructs overlap and can affect each other.

A questionnaire for eudaimonic well-being (QEWB) was developed by Waterman et al. (2010). The QEWB consists of 21 items which build a single common factor.

1.2.4 Flourishing

Psychological well-being as defined by Ryff integrates various approaches from different theoretical backgrounds, but there are some approaches which go even further and consider a more general concept than psychological well-being, for example the concept of *flourishing* developed by Keyes et al. (2002) and Keyes (2005).

Four different conceptualizations and operational definitions of flourishing are currently used within the psychological literature: Keyes et al. (2002) and Keyes (2005), Huppert and So (2009, 2013), Diener et al. (2010), and Seligman (2011).

For a detailed comparison of these approaches and empirical data, cf. Hone et al. (2014).

Keyes' approach is derived by examining the Diagnostic and Statistical Manual of Mental Disorders (DSM) identifying each symptom's opposite. Following Keyes, complete mental health can be seen as a combination of high levels of emotional, psychological and social well-being labeled as flourishing.

Huppert and So's conceptual definition of flourishing is grounded upon three factors of well-being: positive characteristics, positive functioning and positive appraisal.

Seligman's conceptual definition of flourishing is based on five well-being components that can be defined and measured as separate but correlated constructs. According to Seligman's interpretation, well-being requires high levels of positive emotions, engagement, positive relationships, meaning and accomplishments. The combination of these components constitutes the construct PERMA which can be measured with the PERMA-Profiler. In addition to that, Seligman outlines and defines flourishing as the "gold-standard" for measuring well-being and emphasizes the increase of flourishing as the main objective of positive psychology.

These four research teams have operationalized flourishing differently, but do all agree on three matters: first, flourishing is derived on a theoretical basis; second, flourishing refers to high levels of subjective well-being; and third, well-being is a multi-dimensional construct that cannot be measured adequately using a single-item assessment.

We regard the concepts of flourishing as generalization of well-being and especially psychological well-being. In all these four conceptualizations, well-being is measured mainly as a feeling, like in Keyes' instrument ("During the past month, how often do you feel…") and Huppert and So's instrument ("Most of the day I feel a sense of accomplishment from what I do"). Accordingly, Diener et al. phrase "I am a good person and live a good life" and Seligman "In general, how often do you feel joyful?" This justifies our approach to see flourishing as well-being and therefore as a criterion for ways to happiness. But especially the questionnaires of Diener et al. and Seligman also give hints for ways to increase well-being (e.g. Seligman: "How often do you achieve important goals you have set for yourself?") If someone tries to achieve self-set goals he is utilizing a good strategy to achieve happiness.

To sum up, depending on the kind of goal, one can derive assumptions about the way to achieve this goal: Pursuing the goal of subjective well-being, the way seems to be not very clear, whereas psychological well-being inspires you to accept yourself, to look for good relationships, lead a self-determined way of life etc., and eudaimonic well-being advocates to engage in activities and to let people work out their abilities. It can be concluded that the kind of goals set for leading a good life gives hints how to achieve it, but they are not very precise. Especially if one is interested in enhancing chances of leading a good life, one needs more detailed information about what people already do or do not do.

1.3 Research to Ways of Living a Good Life

As was mentioned in the introduction, ways for leading a good life were thought of and discussed since ancient times and therefore there are already creative ideas and profound research with respect to the ways of leading a good life.

1.3.1 Veenhoven's Classic Views

Veenhoven (2014) has presented a categorization of classic views on ways to happiness. Interestingly, he uses information from the large World Database of Happiness (Veenhoven 2009) and computes correlations between indicators of the way to happiness and measures of happiness.

Classical teachings on happiness deal with how to live a good life, for which he gives five strands of advice: the way of warrior, the merchant, the philosopher, the peasant and the monk (s. Table 1.2).

In short, the analyses led to the results that the ways of warrior and merchant show positive relationships to happiness, the way of the philosopher shows no relationship and the ways of peasant and the monk show negative relationships with happiness. Although this categorization is more adhoc and may be somewhat arbitrary, it shows results can differ depending on the kind of way. The ways focused on the inner self seem to be ineffective.

1.3.2 Wisdom

The concept of *wisdom* is regarded as way to achieve happiness (Kekes 1983). Wisdom was intensively studied by philosophers of ancient Greece as well as

Table 1.2 Classic ways to happiness following Veenhoven (2014)

Way	Characteristic	Results of analyses
Way of the warrior	This kind of advice is to live a brave and adventurous life, accompanied by fame and power	+
Way of the merchant	Seek success in trading and gain wealth	+
Way of the philosopher	The advice is to live a contemplative life. Happiness is sought in knowledge	0
Way of peasant	The idea is to live a simple life, at best in the country with contact to nature	−
Way of monk	The advice is to live a life of a monk in order to seek refuge behind the walls of a cloister	−

Note: Correlations between special ways to happiness and measures of happiness. +, 0, −: positive, zero or negative relationship

modern philosophers, and also from a psychological point of view. The Berlin Wisdom research group defined wisdom as "ways and means of planning, managing, and understanding a good life" (Baltes and Staudinger 2000, p. 124) and they discriminated five criteria of wisdom: factual and procedural knowledge, and three other criteria: life-span-contextualism, relativism of values and recognition and management of uncertainty. Life-span contextualism means that people have to consider life problems in relation to the domains of life and take them in a lifespan perspective. Relativism of values means that different people could have different values and they have to be tolerated and finally, uncertainty means that one should keep in mind that decisions cannot be made with 100 % certainty and that a lot of factors could play a role, and one has not always the knowledge to make the decisions which afterwards turn out to be correct.

The researchers of the Berlin wisdom group were especially interested in predicting the behavior of wise people, e.g., if wise people were able to counsel other people or if they could reflect their own life in a sophisticated way. This approach of general wisdom concentrated more on cognitive aspects (knowledge) than on emotional and motivational ones. There are other approaches to wisdom which aim to reflect personal wisdom and which try to use performance measures (cf. Staudinger and Gluck 2011). For other concepts of wisdom see Ardelt (2004) and Sternberg (2009).

1.3.3 Self-Determination Theory (SDT)

The Self-determination theory (SDT) offers another class of ways for how to achieve happiness (s. Ryan and Deci 2000; for a summary Baumgardner and Crothers 2010). The main idea of SDT is: If certain basic needs are fulfilled, then happiness and well-being can be the result. These basic needs are autonomy, competence and relatedness. Autonomy needs deal with activities that are self-chosen by the individual and done because the individuals want to do them. In contrast to autonomous activities are those which were imposed by others. Competence needs are fulfilled if one can show behavior that leads to desired results and lets us feel we have abilities. The need of relatedness is fulfilled if social communication leads to support and understanding. There is a lot of research demonstrating clearly the relation between the fulfillment of these basic needs and well-being (cf. Ryan and Deci 2000). Ryan et al. (2013) derive a perspective of SDT on eudaimonia (cf. below). Eudaimonic living can be characterized in terms of four motivational components: (1) pursuing intrinsic goals rather than extrinsic goals; (2) behaving in autonomous rather than controlled way; (3) being mindful and (4) behaving in a way that the afore mentioned basic psychological needs are satisfied. Interestingly, they see the eudaimonic approach not as outcome but as way to happiness.

1.3.4 Strengths and Virtues

Peterson and Seligman (2004, p. 4) tried to classify the virtues and ways leading to a good life: "…what is right about people and specifically about the strengths of character that make the good life possible." The idea was to build a positive analogon to the Diagnostic and Statistical Manual of Mental Disorders (DSM) and the international Classification of Diseases (ICD). One result was the Values in Action Inventory of Strengths (VIA-IS) classification system of virtues and strength, combining 6 virtues and 24 strengths, measured with 240 items, ten items for each character strength.

Therefore, an important modern way to achieve happiness is to live a life full of virtues and to use one's strengths, especially to use one's signature strengths represented by those scales on which particularly high VIA-IS scores were obtained. There is a huge amount of literature showing that using one's strengths is related to happiness and well-being (Peterson et al. 2007). Therefore living a life in virtue and using one's strengths may be a plausible way to happiness.

The concept of virtues is related to moral aspects of a good life and not everybody will agree to view it as the ideal solution to achieve happiness. The concept of the VIA tries to integrate philosophical and psychological traditions from all over the world to avoid a cultural bias. The way the VIA was developed was thoroughly, diligent and empirically grounded. The disadvantage of such a development strategy is, that it does not necessarily lead to a unified integrated approach but rather to an additive combination of important concepts. Although the VIA is grouped to second order virtues, factor analytic results of empirical data do not correspond to the theoretically derived second order concepts (Park et al. 2009). Another reason which may cause unwillingness to answer the VIA-IS is its length: 240 items related to 24 strengths and virtues. Although attempts were made to reduce the number of items (Furnham and Lester 2012), the results do not satisfy because the Furnham and Lester instrument contains only one item per strength, which implies that a single strength cannot be measured adequately.

Although virtues and strengths significantly contribute to happiness, there may be other ways which contribute to the way to happiness.

1.3.5 Orientations to Happiness (OTH)

Another approach which tries to summarize and integrate ways to happiness is the orientations to happiness (OTH) (Peterson et al. 2005). The authors discriminate three ways to happiness: through pleasure, through engagement and through meaning. Each of these ways predicts happiness. Notifiable is also that if these three ways are combined that will be leading to the so-called "full life". The full life is characterized by the highest relationship to happiness. OTH seems to be in fact a really good way to integrate the various ways to happiness, but for our purposes they are on a high aggregation level and may not be concrete enough to give practical hints for various strategies to enhance happiness. Therefore, a more elaborated approach might be helpful.

Grimm et al. (2014) tried to figure out what kind of actual behavior was related to OTH: They found that not one specific dominant OTH category was clearly related to happiness but a balanced portfolio of all three OTH.

1.3.6 Conclusion: Research About Ways to Happiness

We referred to important ways of happiness which all make their contribution but from our perspective we are looking for ways which give a good basis for increasing happiness.

Veenhoven's classical ways to happiness are interesting proposals for conceptualizing traditional ways to happiness, but until now the five ways are only preliminary classifications of ways. Also, his empirical analyses are informative but not the optimal way to study because the results depend on the variables of the classification system to be contained in the World data base of happiness. One might want to take into consideration other categories, e.g. the way of wisdom, the way of virtue, the way of meaning, etc.

Since ancient times wisdom is definitely seen as a way to happiness. The psychological approaches with regard to wisdom are promising, but it could be argued that holistic ways to happiness should include more explicitly emotional and motivational parameters in addition to different forms of knowledge.

SDT has proven its high potential in predicting happiness and eudaimonia and also gives hints how happiness can be increased, but for diagnostic purposes a more differentiated system than three predictors could be helpful.

The strengths and virtues approach by Peterson and Seligman (2004) is intensively and thoroughly studied and it was demonstrated that especially the application of strengths in new ways can help to enhance happiness. But the VIA-questionnaire consists of 240 items, and therefore is definitely too long. Its factor structure seems to be unclear (analyses of Park and Peterson (2006) point to a heart and a mind factor). Following the authors, moral components are important parameters for the VIA system.

The OTH is explicitly derived for measuring orientations to happiness. It comprises three basic orientations which are important pathways to happiness. One might wish for an instrument containing more differentiated components (more than three) and components measuring more behavior and strategies, because those could be easily changed and trained.

1.4 Behavior and Strategies to Enhance Well-Being

Until now we looked at criteria for happiness which could give hints on how to achieve happiness. Then we described conceptual ways to happiness like wisdom, need fulfillment and virtues. But there also exists research looking for more direct ways to happiness, e.g. for strategies and behavior to enhance happiness.

1.4.1 Fordyce

Fordyce (1977, 1983) can be seen as precursor of positive psychology. His criteria for becoming a happy person were labeled as "14 happiness fundamentals". Following Fordyce (1983, p. 484) these fundamentals are: (s. Table 1.3).

Fordyce performed intervention studies to enhance the happiness of his students compared to control groups. He summarized the results of seven studies that 81 % of the participants enhanced their happiness and 38 % reported that they were much happier. In the studies of Fordyce many ideas of positive psychology are applied especially following the view that behavior contributes to happiness and well-being.

1.4.2 Happiness Increasing Strategies (HIS)

Tkach and Lyubomirsky (2006) asked 500 students to report general happiness increasing strategies (HIS). The students were asked to rate how often they use each of 66 strategies (which had been collected in a pilot study) to increase or maintain

Table 1.3 14 Happiness fundamentals (following Fordyce 1983)

No.	Fundamentals
1	Become more active
2	Spend more time socializing with others
3	Be productive at meaningful work
4	Become more organized and better at planning
5	Reduce your amount of worrying
6	Lower expectations and aspirations
7	Learn to be more positive and optimistic
8	Become more present oriented
9	Develop a healthier personality
10	Develop a more outgoing and social personality
11	Be yourself
12	Reduce negative feelings and problems
13	Recognize close relationships as critical to happiness
14	Make happiness an important life priority

Table 1.4 Happiness increasing strategies and examples (Tkach and Lyubomirsky 2006)

Factors	Examples
Social affiliation	Helping others
Partying and clubbing	Bars, alcohol
Mental control	Not to think being unhappy
Instrumental goal pursue	Study
Passive leisure	Watching TV
Active leisure	Exercise
Religion	Praying
Direct attempts to be happy	Smile

their happiness. The authors found 8 factors (cf. Table 1.4) which accounted for 52 % of the variance in happiness.

With respect to the PERMA categories meaningful relationships were detected. In addition to direct relationships between HIS and happiness the authors found indications that HIS can mediate between personality and happiness.

1.4.3 Happiness Inducing Behaviors (HIB)

Warner and Vroman (2011) extracted 14 happiness inducing behaviors (HIB, s. Table 1.5) from a list of empirically tested methods of increasing happiness from Lyubomirsky (2007). Healthy eating was added by Warner and Vroman. Participants were asked to indicate how often in the past 2 months they had shown each of the behaviors.

Table 1.5 Happiness inducing behaviors and factors, Warner and Vroman (2011)

	Positive/proactive	Spiritual	Health
Relationships	x		
Kindness	x		
Optimism	x		
Savoring	x		
Goals	x		
New ways to cope	x	x	
Gratitude	x	x	
Flow	x		
Avoiding worry	x		
Religion		x	
Meditation		x	
Forgiveness		x	
Physical exercise			x

Note: x: loading >.30

Factor analysis yielded 3 factors: positive/proactive behavior, spiritual behavior and physical health behavior, which explained 48 % of the variance. The authors also showed that the relationship between personality and happiness is mediated by the HIB (s. Table 1.5).

1.4.4 Meta-Analyses of Interventions of PP

Because interventions of positive psychology (PP) are usually derived to reduce negative feelings and/or enhance positive affect, these interventions contain elements of strategies we are interested in.

A study by Seligman et al. (2005) evaluated the empirical validity of interventions from positive psychology and showed that three of them (good things, gratitude and using signature strengths in a new way) lastingly increased happiness.

Nowadays there are a lot of positive psychology interventions and meta-analyses were performed to test their overall effectiveness, e.g. Sin and Lyubomirsky (2009), who studied 51 interventions, Bolier et al. (2013) and Hone et al. (2014) give a categorization of the studies they included in their meta-analyses. These categories are kind of therapies, gratitude intervention, intervention packages, optimism, coaching, resilience, kindness/compassion, bibliotherapy and mindfulness. Hope and savoring were included within packages.

For our purpose it seems to be important that these categories provide no clear taxonomy for PP interventions but are just adhoc groupings of more superficial aspects of interventions. A more systematic approach stems from Quoidbach et al. (2015) following the perspective of emotion regulation. The categories for PP interventions are spanned by two dimensions, a family of emotion regulation strategies (situation selection, situation modification, attentional deployment, cognitive change, and response modulation), and time frame (before, during and after positive emotional events). Although these categories are very helpful for detecting research deficits, they are not perfectly applicable to all cases, e.g. to positive psychotherapy or coaching which might fit into more than one of the categories.

1.4.5 Conclusion

To sum up, we presented more concrete strategies and behaviors to achieve happiness. But whereas the orientations to happiness (OTH) seemed too general for deriving clear hints what to do for leading a good life, the behaviors and strategies described here are often very specific, e.g., watching TV, going to bars, etc.… and could not be taken as adequate general ways for leading a good life. Although there exist factor analytic reductions for the behaviors and strategies, neither the HIB nor the HIS seem to contain the right level of information and they don't seem to be a profound system which is helpful to give advice for enhancing ways leading a good life. What is needed is a concept which is more concrete than OTH and more general than HIB.

1.5 Our Own Concept: Overview

Our aim is to propose ways to lead a good life. Until now we tried to discriminate between the effects of leading a good life, being different kinds of well-being, and means to achieve well-being, which are strategies and attitudes. The latter are, from our point of view, predictors of well-being. Unfortunately, there are a lot of concepts which do not clearly make this difference between criterion and predictors. An example is psychological well-being which is, as a kind of well-being, the goal to be achieved but also the means to achieve it. For the included construct "purpose in life", one question is: "I live one day at a time and don't really think about the future". If someone lives his or her life in this way, he or she follows a way to achieve a good life, but the PWB is mainly a measure of well-being and therefore intended for measuring the result of leading a good life.

1.5.1 Our Criteria for a Concept for Art-of-Living

We developed our own criteria for our concept of art-of-living and will often be referring to examples which do not meet our criteria to make the point clear. Firstly, we describe the aspects that guided us for the theoretical considerations.

Following the schema of Veenhoven (2013) we discriminate between *means to achieve happiness* and the *result* which may be happiness. Art-of-living is an integrated ensemble of ways to happiness. These means can be conceptualized as strategies or attitudes, for example, to stay in contact with ones friends is a way of behavior.

Furthermore, art-of-living tries to be a *holistic and integrated* concept and therefore does not limit to only one or two ways to achieve happiness but it tries to integrate various aspects regarding the body, the self, the soul and the mind. The strategies of Fordyce (1977, 1983) also compose a variety of different ways to happiness, but they cannot be seen as parameters of an integrative overall concept.

The strategies should *not be too abstract*, e.g. one advice people often get, "be happy", as in the famous song, does not really help, because the main question is definitely: "what can we do to be happy?" But also the strategies should *not be too fine-grained or narrow* like "drink a cup of coffee", because there are numerous ways to shortly enhance mood by taking food or drinks.

Different from the concept of virtues and strengths, art-of-living tries to *avoid being too moralistic:* Whereas Peterson and Seligman (2004, p. 13) explicitly note that "Virtues are the core characteristics valued by moral philosophers and religious thinkers", in art-of-living the moral aspect is only implicitly included, e.g. to have an optimistic attitude towards life is part of the art-of-living concept, because it contributes to a better life and not because an optimistic view is valued as good per se. It is not possible to avoid that the concepts are related to various values but it is not the main intention to prescribe from a moral perspective what is good and what is not.

There is *not only one way of art-of-living* (therefore Veenhoven 2003a, b advocated the notion "arts-of-living") but numerous ways lead to happiness. Therefore, the construct is multidimensional and it integrates many aspects and, in consequence, many pathways to happiness. *Each individual may have its own art-of-living.*

As pointed out in the discrimination between means and results, art-of-living is the mean to be happy, and therefore, the application of its various strategies is supposed to lead to happiness. The concept of art-of-living includes *attitudes and strategies*, which is important insofar, as attitudes and strategies can be changed. One can choose another, more appropriate, strategy if one does not lead to desired outcomes. That does not mean that individuals change their strategies day by day. Strategies have some stability but not as much as stable personality factors. Because art-of-living strategies can be changed, they also can be content of interventions especially derived to enhance art-of-living. Therefore, *Art-of-living can be learnt.*

One central aspect of our research is that *art-of-living can be measured* (different from philosophical considerations). This is also different for some approaches from humanistic psychology which were of great theoretical importance but failed to provide sufficient instruments for the measurement of core constructs (like C.G. Jung (1933) and Maslow (1968)). In the first step, we evaluate if the main ideas of our concept of art-of-living are shared by lay people. Secondly, we develop a *multidimensional instrument* for measuring art-of-living. This instrument is tested with regard to the common criteria of *reliability and validity.* For validation, the nomological network of art-of-living is analyzed with respect to related constructs, among them wisdom, resilience, sense of coherence, self-regulation, Orientations to Happiness, strengths and virtues. Criteria are subjective well-being, psychological well-being, flourishing including PERMA and eudaimonic well-being and (missing) depression.

It is also an empirical question whether our aspects of art-of-living can be viewed as separate dimensions within factor analyses. Following the idea that art-of-living are means to achieve happiness, the core test of our construct is that it is possible to significantly *predict well-being using art-of-living.* It has to be tested if art-of-living, in addition to personality, predicts well-being better than personality alone. And finally, there's need for evaluation if *art-of-living can be trained in intervention studies* for different groups and also, if increased art-of-living leads to increased well-being.

1.5.2 Philosophical Background: Wilhelm Schmid

We now focus on the philosophical background. Wilhelm Schmid (1998, 2004) has written a series of books dealing with the art-of-living. In his book entitled "Philosophie der Lebenskunst" (German for "the philosophy of the art-of-living"), Schmid (1998) reintroduced the art-of-living in German philosophy. He elaborated his ideas in his more recent work "To be friends with ourselves" (Schmid 2004), in which he draws on important concepts by Foucault. Among the main ones is the care for oneself.

We relate to some important ideas from Schmid from which we draw in the following. What is meant by art of living? Schmid (2004, p. 9) describes the scope of his concept of art-of-living in the following way: "Art-of-living is not meant as the easy, happy-go-lucky life but the conscious, reflected conduct of life." Therefore, it can cost great efforts as well as be a special source of fulfillment.

Why using the term *art?* According to Schmid, art refers to a challenge as well as a high quality of doing something. Art is meant with respect to high competence and the will to perform excellent. Art-of-living is related to the process of living and not a final product to be achieved.

The concept art-of-living dates back to ancient terms like the Greek *téchnē tou biou* or the Latin *ars vitae* or *ars vivendi* (Nehamas 1998) and is seen in line with Sokrates' and Platon's understanding of the term as care for oneself (Nehamas 1998). The art-of-living deals with a modest relationship of the individual to itself, which allows strengthening the self and an opening to others. The self gives itself structure and form and makes life a work of art. Working on the self also enables the construction of meaning. Dealing with art of living cannot give normative rules how to live but it can offer options how to proceed in life. The forming of life includes high investment of effort, and savoring cannot be the only way to happiness. The forming of life is an individual undertaking. Reflection on one's life includes thinking about fundamental questions like *What is the meaning of life? What is a good life? Am I on the right way? What is the meaning of pain, death, sickness? What are important values for me?* and *What is happiness?* Thinking about these questions does not necessarily mean one finds final answers, but may be priorities for one's different values, a differentiated knowledge about oneself and a way of living one's life with more care.

A sentence at the entrance of the Greek temple of Delphi "gnōthi sautón" "know thyself" emphasizes the importance of self-knowledge. To be an artist-of-living, self-knowledge is the precondition for a good life, but it is also important to live one's own life, which means to follow one's own laws, which is the original meaning of being autonomous.

In sum, according to Schmid, main attributes of the art-of-living are to live a conscious, effortful, self-determined, competent, reflective way of life.

Succeeding a long tradition in philosophy, Schmid relates art-of-living to the following aspects of the human being: the body, the soul and the mind. Schmid has written a lot on the topic, we can only select some aspects which seem to be important from our perspective.

1.5.2.1 Body

Clearly, a good life depends on a good physical condition. According to the idea of positive psychology for the body, it is not sufficient for a good life not to be sick, but healthy in a positive way, meaning one feels active, energetic, etc. Ways to influence that are nutrition, exercise and the use of the five senses. In typical intervention programs of positive psychology savoring is included, which often recommends using the five senses intensively.

1.5.2.2 Soul

In philosophy the concept of the soul is still in use whereas, at present, in psychology the concept of soul is not referred to, but some related topics are dealt with within the scope of emotion. The art-of-living includes both positive emotions, but also grief, anxiety, and pain. It can especially unfold in difficult situations when individuals have to cope with the ups and downs, the hassles and problems of everyday life. Schmid refers to the necessity of emotion regulation to live a good life, which, from our perspective, we would categorize as coping strategies. Schmid also underlines the need for finding a balance between extreme emotional states, e.g. enthusiastically expressing negative emotions or suppressing any kind of emotion.

1.5.2.3 Mind

With respect to the mind, art-of-living is characterized by a reflective way of living, knowing oneself, and an active striving for one's goals. Schmid refers to various kinds of writing as ways to reflect on one's life, e.g. in the form of diaries or what psychologists would term expressive writing (Pennebaker 1997). Regarding the experiencing of various life events, he advocates as mental strategy to stay as even-tempered as possible. Schmid (1998) argues that a generally positive attitude towards life and the world, openness to what life might present, and some kind of serenity might be helpful in the ups and downs of life. Finally, it is important to find some meaning in life.

Although the self plays an important role in Schmid's theory of the art-of-living, the concept is not restricted to self-attention. The forming of the environment and the importance of healthy and strong relationships with others are also important.

Different from the field of philosophy, the topic of the art-of-living has not been discussed or investigated much in the field of psychology. There is no consistent definition or operationalization, and very little research concerning the construct of art-of-living exists so far. However, related topics such as happiness, well-being, quality of life, resilience, a sense of coherence, and wisdom have been studied to a greater degree (see Sect. 1.3).

1.5.3 Our Model of the Art-of-Living

In the introduction to the special issue of the Journal of happiness studies, Veenhoven (2003a) states that the art-of-living may be an appropriate venue for intervention. He believes that the art-of-living consists of skills that, to some extent, can be learned (Veenhoven 2003a). We share this opinion and work to address the question which aspects and skills are included in the art-of-living and how they can be measured. Therefore, we created and evaluated a questionnaire that measures an individual's extent of the art-of-living. In addition to the empirical results, the liberal model of the art-of-living by Schmid (1998, 2004) formed the background. Accordingly, we discuss the following basic concepts of our model.

Transferring Schmid's (1998, 2004) concept into a psychological model as the basis of a questionnaire was quite difficult for different reasons. Firstly, philosophical concepts are far from being easily measurable because measurement is not the primary intention of a philosophical author. Secondly, in Schmid's theory, there is a broad overlap between some concepts (e.g., caring for the self can happen at the level of the body, soul, or mind). Thirdly, the concepts and strategies of the art-of-living are very rich and broad (e.g., bodily care can include dancing, singing, exercising, using one's senses, etc.). Therefore, it is difficult to select the most important ones from this broad list of concepts. In sum, we were confronted with at least three problems: the question of measurability of the concepts, the question of concept overlap, and finally, the question of completeness. Another question was whether the selected psychological concepts were able to capture the richness of the philosophical concepts. We will provide preliminary empirical solutions to all of these questions. First, we try to show that our instrument contains components that fulfill the usual measurement criteria. Second, we try to show that the concepts, although there might be substantial overlap, have different specificity by computing correlations and factor analyses. Third, using correlations and factor analyses, we try to illustrate that the group of components show sufficient communality so that it makes sense to talk about a general concept called the art-of-living. Fourth, by predicting happiness by art-of-living we will show that art-of-living can substantially contribute to happiness. Fifth, the question of the predictive power of these components is tested via regression analyses. We also try to demonstrate that art-of-living can add to personality as we use regression analyses and include personality variables as a first step and then add art-of-living to the equation. Finally, it is an empirical question if other researchers may substitute variables or add more variables that will enhance the predictive power.

The four chapters of Schmid's (2004) book can be used as the main categories for our model: care of the self, the body, the soul, and the mind. We extracted one more category, environment, which seems to be important from a psychological perspective. Namely, (a) good contact with other people and (b) the shaping of living conditions, are both subsumed under this additional level. In the following, the subcategories are listed with a short description of each of the main categories.

- Self-care:
  - *A self-determined way of living* (setting one's own goals and seeing meaning in life)
  - *Self-efficacy* (being able to deal with difficult situations and problems)
  - *Self-knowledge* (knowing one's own strengths and weaknesses)
- Bodily care
  - *Physical self-caring* (caring for the well-being of the body; e.g., through physical exercise)
  - *Savoring* (doing something one likes and savor it)
- Care of the soul (the soul is related to emotion and motivation)
  - *Balance* (finding a balance between different emotions as well as emotions and cognitions)
  - *Integrating different areas of living* (living a flexible work-life balance)
  - *Coping* (being able to cope also with unpleasant events)
- Care of the mind (in psychological terminology, care of the mind is related to cognition)
  - *Positive attitude towards life* (having a positive orientation toward life)
  - *Serenity* (keeping calm even in difficult situations)
  - *Openness* (being open to new developments in one's life and the world)
  - *Optimization* (trying to get good results and trying to become better)
- Environment
  - *Social contact* (trying to have good relationships with other people)
  - *Shaping of living conditions* (trying to form one's environment following one's goals; e.g., home)

Because balance is not as widely used as other concepts, we refer to Sternberg's (2009) wisdom model, which incorporates balance as main component. Sirgy and Wu (2013) also relate the balanced life to well-being, but use it mainly in the sense of balance of different life domains and it is more related to our *integrating different areas of living*.

1.6 Summary and Conclusion

After this introduction to the components of our model, we summarize important aspects of the construct art-of-living. First, we understand art-of-living not as the outcome of leading a good life but as a predictor of it. We have to demonstrate that empirically: *art-of-living can significantly predict well-being*. Art-of-living can contribute to happiness and well-being, but it is distinct from these concepts. Second, art-of-living will be conceptualized *not too general, not too fine-grained and not too moralistic*. Third, following Veenhoven (2003a, b), we argue that art-of-living can be performed *in many different ways* and each individual can find its own way. Fourth, art-of-living includes *strategies as well as attitudes*. Fifth, we consider that the *art-of-living can be learned* and especially certain aspects of it. That means, *art-of-living can be realized by almost everyone* and not only by experts (like philosophers or artists). Sixth, we want to show that *art-of-living can be measured with reliability and validity*. Seventh, we demonstrate *empirically that we can design interventions that can enhance art-of-living and happiness* for different groups.

References

Andrew, F. M., & Withey, S. B. (1976). *Social indicators of well-being* (pp. 20–31). New York and London: Plenum.

Ardelt, M. (2004). Wisdom as expert knowledge system: A critical review of a contemporary operationalization of an ancient concept. *Human Development, 47*(5), 257–285.

Baltes, P. B., & Staudinger, U. M. (2000). Wisdom: A metaheuristic (pragmatic) to orchestrate mind and virtue toward excellence. *American Psychologist, 55*(1), 122–136.

Baumgardner, S. R., & Crothers, M. K. (2010). *Positive psychology*. Upper Saddle River, NJ: Pearson.

Bolier, L., Haverman, M., Westerhof, G. J., Riper, H., Smit, F., & Bohlmeijer, E. (2013). Positive psychology interventions: A meta-analysis of randomized controlled studies. *BMC Public Health, 13*(1), 119.

Diener, E. (1984). Subjective well-being. *Psychological Bulletin, 95*, 542–575.

Diener, E. D., Emmons, R. A., Larsen, R. J., & Griffin, S. (1985). The satisfaction with life scale. *Journal of Personality Assessment, 49*(1), 71–75.

Diener, E., Ng, W., Harter, J., & Arora, R. (2010). Wealth and happiness across the world: material prosperity predicts life evaluation, whereas psychosocial prosperity predicts positive feeling. *Journal of Personality and Social Psychology, 99*(1), 52–61.

Diener, E., & Lucas, R. E. (1999). Personality and subjective well-being. In D. Kahneman, E. Diener, & N. Schwarz (Eds.), *Well-being: Foundations of hedonic psychology* (pp. 213–229). New York: Russell Sage Foundation.

Erikson, E. H. (1959). Identity and the life cycle. *Psychological Issues, 1*, 50–100.

Fordyce, M. (1977). Development of a program to increase personal happiness. *Journal of Counseling Psychology, 24*(6), 511–521.

Fordyce, M. (1983). A program to increase happiness: further studies. *Journal of Counseling Psychology, 30*(4), 483–498.

Furnham, A., & Lester, D. (2012). The development of a short measure of character strength. *European Journal of Psychological Assessment, 28*, 95–101.

Grimm, C., Kemp, S., & Jose, P. E. (2014). Orientations to happiness and the experience of everyday activities. *The Journal of Positive Psychology, 10*(3), 207–218.

Hone, L. C., Jarden, A., Schofield, G. M., & Duncan, S. (2014). Measuring flourishing: The impact of operational definitions on the prevalence of high levels of wellbeing. *International Journal of Wellbeing, 4*(1), 62–90.

Huppert, F. A., & So, T. (2009). What percentage of people in Europe are flourishing and what characterises them. In *IX ISQOLS conference*.

Huppert, F. A., & So, T. T. (2013). Flourishing across Europe: Application of a new conceptual framework for defining well-being. *Social Indicators Research, 110*(3), 837–861.

Huta, V., & Waterman, A. S. (2014). Eudaimonia and its distinction from hedonia: Developing a classification and terminology for understanding conceptual and operational definitions. *Journal of Happiness Studies, 15*(6), 1425–1456.

Jung, C. G. (1933). *Modern man in search of a soul*. New York: Harcourt & Brace.

Kekes, J. (1983). Wisdom. *American Philosophical Quarterly, 20*(3), 277–286.

Keyes, C. L. (2005). Mental illness and/or mental health? Investigating axioms of the complete state model of health. *Journal of Consulting and Clinical Psychology, 73*(3), 539–548.

Keyes, C., Shmotkin, D. & Ryff, C. (2002). Optimizing well-being: The empirical encounter of two traditions. *Journal of Personality and Social Psychology, 82*, 1007–1022.

Lyubomirsky, S. (2007). *The how of happiness: A new approach to getting the life you want*. London: Penguin.

Lyubomirsky, S. (2008). *The how of happiness: A scientific approach to getting the life you want*. New York: Penguin.

Maslow, A. H. (1968). *Toward a psychology of being* (2nd ed.). New York: Van Nostrand.

Michalos, A. C. (2015). *Ancient views on the quality of life*. New York: Springer.

Nehamas, A. (1998). *The art of living: Socratic reflections from Plato to Foucault* (Vol. 61). California: University of California Press.

Park, N., & Peterson, C. (2006). Moral competence and character strengths among adolescents: The development and validation of the values in action inventory of strengths for youth. *Journal of adolescence, 29*(6), 891–909.

Park, N., Peterson, C., & Ruch, W. (2009). Orientations to happiness and life satisfaction in twenty-seven nations. *The Journal of Positive Psychology, 4*(4), 273–279.

Pennebaker, J. W. (1997). Writing about emotional experiences as a therapeutic process. *Psychological Science, 8*(3), 162–166.

Peterson, C., & Seligman, M. E. P. (2004). *Character strengths and virtues: A handbook and classification*. Oxford: Oxford University Press.

Peterson, C., Park, N., & Seligman, M. E. P. (2005). Orientations to happiness and life satisfaction: the full life versus the empty life. *Journal of Happiness Studies, 6*(1), 25–41.

Peterson, C., Ruch, W., Beermann, U., Park, N., & Seligman, M. E. P. (2007). Strength of character, orientations to happiness, and life satisfaction. *The Journal of Positive Psychology, 2*(3), 149–156.

Quoidbach, J., Mikolajczak, M., & Gross, J. J. (2015). Positive interventions: An emotion regulation perspective. *Psychological Bulletin, 141*(3), 655–693.

Rogers, C. R. (1961). *On becoming a person*. Boston: Houghton Mifflin.

Ryan, R. M., & Deci, E. L. (2000). Self-determination theory and the facilitation of intrinsic motivation, social development, and well-being. *American Psychologist, 55*(1), 68–78.

Ryan, R. M., Huta, V., & Deci, E. L. (2013). Living well: A self-determination theory perspective on eudaimonia. In *The exploration of happiness* (pp. 117–139). Netherlands: Springer.

Ryff, C. D. (1989). Happiness is everything, or is it? Explorations on the meaning of psychological well-being. *Journal of Personality and Social Psychology, 57*(6), 1069–1081.

Ryff, C. D., & Singer, B. (1996). Psychological well-being: Meaning, measurement, and implications for psychotherapy research. *Psychotherapy and Psychosomatics, 65*(1), 14–23.

Schmid, W. (1998). *Philosophie der Lebenskunst: Eine Grundlegung*. Frankfurt am Main: Suhrkamp Publishers.

Schmid, W. (2004). *Mit sich befreundet sein. Von der Lebenskunst im Umgang mit sich selbst*. Frankfurt am Main: Suhrkamp Publishers.

Seligman, M. E., Steen, T. A., Park, N., & Peterson, C. (2005). Positive psychology progress: Empirical validation of interventions. *American Psychologist, 60*(5), 410–421.

Seligman, M. E. P. (2011). *Flourish: A visionary new understanding of happiness and well-being*. New York: Free Press.

Sin, N. L., & Lyubomirsky, S. (2009). Enhancing well-being and alleviating depressive symptoms with positive psychology interventions: A practice-friendly meta-analysis. *Journal of Clinical Psychology, 65*(5), 467–487.

Sirgy, M. J., & Wu, J. (2013). The pleasant life, the engaged life, and the meaningful life: what about the balanced life? In *The exploration of happiness* (pp. 175–191). Netherlands: Springer.

Staudinger, U. M., & Gluck, J. (2011). Psychological wisdom research: Commonalities and differences in a growing field. *Annual Review of Psychology, 62*, 215–241.

Sternberg, R. J. (2009). Wisdom, intelligence & creativity synthesized. *School Administrator, 66*(2), 10–11.

Tkach, C., & Lyubomirsky, S. (2006). How do people pursue happiness? Relating personality, happiness-increasing strategies, and well-being. *Journal of Happiness Studies, 7*(2), 183–225.

Veenhoven, R. (2003a). Arts-of-living. *Journal of Happiness Studies, 4*, 373–384.

Veenhoven, R. (2003b). Notions of art-of-living. *Journal of Happiness Studies, 4*(4), 345–349.

Veenhoven, R. (2009). World database of happiness. *Psychological Topics, 18*, 221–246.

Veenhoven, R. (2013). The four qualities of life ordering concepts and measures of the good life. In Delle Fave, A. (Ed.), *The Exploration of Happiness: Present and future Perpectives* (pp. 195–226). Dodrecht, Netherlands: Springer.

Veenhoven, R. (2014). Classic wisdom about ways to happiness: How does it apply today? In *The pursuit of happiness and the traditions of wisdom* (pp. 1–12). Netherlands: Springer.

Warner, R. M., & Vroman, K. G. (2011). Happiness inducing behaviors in everyday life: An empirical assessment of "the how of happiness". *Journal of Happiness Studies, 12*(6), 1063–1082. doi:10.1007/s10902-010-9245-3.

Waterman, A. S. (1990). The relevance of Aristotle's conception of eudaimonia for the psychological study of happiness. *Theoretical & Philosophical Psychology, 10*(1), 39–44. doi:10.1037/h0091489.

Waterman, A. S., Schwartz, S. J., Zamboanga, B. L., Ravert, R. D., Williams, M. K., Bede Agocha, V., et al. (2010). The questionnaire for eudaimonic well-being: Psychometric properties, demographic comparisons, and evidence of validity. *The Journal of Positive Psychology, 5*(1), 41–61. doi:10.1080/17439760903435208.

Chapter 2
Development of a Questionnaire Measuring Art-of-Living

2.1 Introduction

2.1.1 Questions Regarding the Concept

Firstly, we perform a study aiming to investigate how people think about art-of-living: Are their opinions similar to the ones we phrased in the introduction? Do they believe that art-of-living can be learnt? Do they see a way to perform art-of-living? To answer these questions, in this study we were asking open- as well as closed questions regarding the concept of art-of-living.

To be precise, our research questions regarding the concept are:

1. What opinions do people have regarding art-of-living? Are they similar to the concepts developed by Wilhelm Schmid?
2. Do people think that art-of-living can be learned?
3. Do people think there is only one way to perform art-of-living?
4. Are there different types of artists of living?

2.1.2 Questions Regarding the Instrument and Its Validity, Reliability and Factorial Structure

Secondly, we derive a multidimensional questionnaire based on the survey results. We want to test the quality of this instrument by computing internal consistency, extracting the factorial structure and trying to validate it. To achieve this, we also used life-satisfaction as one criterion variable. Therefore, our research questions regarding the instrument are:

5. Can a reliable questionnaire with corresponding sub-constructs be developed for art-of-living?

B. Schmitz, *Art-of-Living*, Social Indicators Research Series 63,
DOI 10.1007/978-3-319-45324-8_2

6. Can the factorial structure of the subscales be reproduced adequately?
7. Is there a general factor model underlying the whole instrument?
8. Is our questionnaire measuring art-of-living sufficiently free from effects of social desirability?
9. Can art-of-living be used to predict happiness?

2.1.3 *Sequence of Studies*

This chapter describes four studies. In Study 1, a preliminary questionnaire consisting of a mixture of open (five) and closed (six) questions was used in order to analyze qualitatively and quantitatively whether our conceptions of art-of-living are similar to the conceptions held in our sample (N = 128). In a pilot study for study 2, we pretested our newly developed questionnaire for our 14 sub-constructs to a pilot sample (N = 65). On the basis of this data, some of the items were modified. This version of the questionnaire was then used in our main Study 2 with a sample of N = 1105.

Findings were discussed and complemented by theoretical and our own considerations in order to create the questionnaire. The resulting version contains 14 scales, which measure the different components of art-of-living.

The next step in Study 3 is to improve the questionnaire both from a theoretical and an empirical basis. Finally we discuss in Study 4 a short form of the questionnaire for application in contexts which do not allow the usage of the complete questionnaire.

2.2 Study 1: Preliminary Combined Qualitative and Quantitative Survey: How Do People Think About Art-of-Living?

Anna Schmidt

2.2.1 *Method Study 1*

The purpose of the preliminary interview was to find out whether our conceptions of art-of-living were shared in our sample. In order to compare our theoretical considerations with common views, we asked our sample about their ideas concerning art-of-living. Furthermore, to obtain qualitative data we posed six open questions concerning art-of-living (see Table 2.1). For gaining quantitative data we asked four questions in a closed answer format (see Table 2.2). The answers to these questions served as an additional source for developing and phrasing the final questionnaire.

Table 2.1 Open questions in the preliminary interview with exemplary answers

Question	Exemplary answer
What do you understand art-of-living to mean?	To find solutions that contribute to personal satisfaction even in difficult situations Art-of-living is to make the best out of what you have and to be happy with that/it
Which traits would you ascribe to a life artist?	Inner strengths, strong-mindedness, creativity serenity, courage
What does being a life-artist bring with it?	Serenity, satisfaction, to feel happiness in life Not to become desperate
How can art-of-living be seen in your life?	To accept day-to-day circumstances and practice serenity Creativity and improvisation
How can you bring more art-of-living into your life?	Enjoy the moment and do not get tangled up in worries about the future In not being too perfectionistic To seek new ideas and goals and fulfill them
Do you know someone who practices art-of-living? If yes, what characterizes this individual?	Independent of the opinion of others, strong personality, committed to his/her own thing

Table 2.2 Closed questions in the preliminary interview and their quantities in the responses

Item	Quantity (%)
For art-of-living you need	
Talent	16.4
Routine	29.7
Experience	36
Certain personality traits	58.6
A balance between activity and passivity	42.2
Art-of-living is	
A deliberate/conscious way of living	47.7
Desirable	37.5
Accepting things that happen	42.2
Different for each individual	49.2
Appreciating life′s little pleasures	46.9
Do you associate the term life-artist with something positive or negative?	
Positive	78.9
Negative	21.1
Art-of-living is reserved for the few people who were born as life-artists?	
Yes	18
No	68
Missings	14.1

The preliminary interview was filled out by 128 participants and completed by 92 participants. The mean age was 35 with a range of 19–79 years; about 32 % of the participants were male and about 41 % were female (27 % did not specify); as to the sample's occupation, 50 % of the participants were students, 35.9 % had a university degree, 9.8 % had a qualified job, and 4.3 % were graduates.

Table 2.1 shows the open questions with which the participants were asked to write down their personal opinions regarding art-of-living and life-artists. In order to organize and sum the answers to the open questions, a set of categories was developed. Based on the different components that were mentioned by the participants, 11 categories were generated inductively to classify the answers.

2.2.2 *Results of Study 1*

2.2.2.1 Research Question 1, 2, 3

Table 2.3 contains the 11 categories. The answers were assigned to one or several of the categories (depending on the components that were mentioned). To ensure objectivity, the classification was conducted independently by several members of the research team (Bortz and Döring 2006). Table 2.3 also lists how many answers (from all open questions) were assigned to each category. The answer to the question "What do you understand by art-of-living?" was, for example, assigned to categories one and nine: *"To be able to accommodate to the different phases and problems of life and to gain positive strengths by these situations. Good balance between work and free time."*

Most answers (i.e., over 65 %) were assigned to the first three categories. These answers connected art-of-living to a successful handling of negative events, optimism, and a positive attitude toward life as well as a self-determined way of living.

Table 2.3 Description of empirical categories and frequencies of their answers

No.	Category	Frequencies of answers	Percentages of answers (%)
1	Handling of negative events, optimism, positive attitude towards life, humor	222	33.8
3	Self-determined way of living	127	19.3
2	Creativity, openness	104	15.8
6	Satisfaction with one's current state	41	6.2
5	Serenity	40	6.1
4	Deliberate exploration of pleasant activities	37	5.6
10	Relationships, social contact	22	3.3
7	Pragmatism/efficiency	19	2.9
9	Balance	19	2.9
8	Emphasis on the present	17	2.6
11	Reflection	9	1.4

Furthermore, art-of-living was described by many participants with openness and creativity.

Five items were framed in a closed format (see Table 2.2). They related to the concepts people have regarding the conditions for art-of-living, whether it is individual, positive, reserved for few people, and, whether it is mainly a topic for philosophers. For Items 1 and 2, the participants could choose multiple options (1 to all). Frequencies of the different answer options are shown in Table 2.2.

The evaluation of the closed questions shows that most participants connected the term life-artist' to something positive. Predominantly, they did not think that art-of-living is reserved for natural born life-artists or lies only in the interest of philosophers. The statement "For art-of-living, you need" was completed most frequently by "certain personality traits", followed by the statement "For art-of-living, you need a balance between activity and passivity." The alternatives "For art-of-living, you need experience" and "For art-of-living, you need routine" were chosen less often. The least approval was obtained for the answer "For art-of-living, you need talent." The statement "art-of-living is" could likewise be completed by different answers. For this statement, the different reply options were chosen more or less equally often. Thus, art-of-living is seen as a deliberate/conscious way of living, it is seen as desirable, as accepting of things that happen, as different for each individual, and as appreciating life's little pleasures.

In sum, it can be stated that this sample considers art-of-living to be something positive and desirable. The participants see art-of-living as learnable but facilitated by certain personality traits. They connect art-of-living mainly with a satisfying and successful life even when facing negative events and a way of living that is determined by the individual's wishes, ideas, and ideals. Furthermore, art-of-living and especially the life-artist are characterized by creativity and openness.

2.3 Study 2: The Questionnaire Measuring Art-of-Living

Anna Schmidt

2.3.1 Method of Study 2

2.3.1.1 Art-of-Living Questionnaire

For generating the art-of-living-questionnaire, 14 scales and corresponding items were generated. Thereby, the categories from the preliminary interview were taken into account, adapted and supplemented based on relevant literature and our own theoretical considerations, at which the components of art-of-living according to Schmid (2004) were considered in particular. In addition, as we consider self-efficacy to be a relevant component of art-of-living, we also included the

Table 2.4 Demographic characteristics of pilot sample and main sample

	Pilot sample ($N = 64$) (%)	Main sample ($N = 1105$) (%)
Age (years)		
13–20	3.1	9.5
21–24	12.8	25.7
25–34	56.3	30.6
35–44	11	12.9
45–54	6.3	12.8
55–64	9.4	5.7
65+	1.6	3.4
Sex		
Male	27.6	34.8
Female	56.6	65.2
Missing	15.8	
Family/relationship status		
Single	21.1	30.4
In a relationship	40.8	42.2
Married	21.1	22.3
Divorced	1.3	4.2
Widowed	–	1
Children		
Yes	19.7	24.8
No	64.5	75.2
Education		
High school	2.6	10.4
Professional education	11.8	12.2
High school graduate	36.8	46.3
University degree	32.9	33.9
Nationality		
European	100	98.2
American	–	.54
Asian	–	.81
n.s.	–	.45

general self-efficacy scale by Schwarzer and Jerusalem (Hinz et al. 2006), which is an established instrument with valid psychometric properties (Hinz et al. 2006).

A pilot sample ($N = 64$) was asked to fill out the questionnaire so that psychometric properties could be assessed. The demographic characteristics of the pilot sample are summarized in a column of Table 2.4.

Most scales showed satisfactory internal consistencies ranging from $\alpha = .65$ to $\alpha = .89$. The internal consistency of the questionnaire as whole was .92. The internal consistencies of the scales *coping* and *shaping of living conditions* were rather low at first, that is why some items were removed or rephrased to improve internal consistencies.

2.3.1.2 Sample

The sample was recruited on the basis of an online questionnaire. Table 2.4 (right column) summarizes the demographic characteristics of the sample.

The participants were mainly of German nationality with only a few other nationalities. The total sample consisted of 1105 people.

Table 2.5 lists the final subscales with one exemplary item. The participants were asked to answer each item on a 6-point scale depending on the extent the statement applied to them (1 = *does not apply at all* to 6 = *totally applies*). The questionnaire also encompassed the following demographic data: sex, age, nationality, highest level of education, occupational status (e.g., employee, executive), family/relationship status and children. Furthermore, the questionnaire included a question concerning the participants' religiousness/spirituality. To find out about the participants' view on the learnability of art-of-living, we also asked the participants whether they assume that art-of-living can be learned and whether they agree/disagree with the statement "There is only one way to live a fulfilling life."

2.3.1.3 Measures for Validation

Satisfaction with Life Scale (SWLS)

The Satisfaction with Life Scale (Diener et al. 1985) was included in the final questionnaire in order to record satisfaction with life as a criterion variable.

Table 2.5 Final subscales of the questionnaire with exemplary items

No.	Final subscale	Exemplary item
1	Coping	I arise strengthened from painful experiences
2	Openness	I like to take on new challenges
3	Self-determined way of living	I work toward realizing my personal goals
4	Savoring	I spoil myself
5	Serenity	I do not easily get worked up
6	Integrating different areas of living	I take enough time for my hobbies
7	Balance	I can not only plan very well but also intuitively approach a task
8	Social contact	I know people with whom I can be who I am
9	Self-knowledge	I know my own strengths and weaknesses
10	Physical care	I pay attention to my body
11	Optimization	I arrange my strengths quite well
12	Positive attitude towards life	Altogether, I expect that I will experience more good than bad things
13	Self-efficacy	For every problem, I can find a solution
14	Shaping of living conditions	In my accommodation/home, I feel comfortable

The SWLS measures an individual's evaluation of satisfaction with life in general. Previous research has reported good psychometric properties for the SWLS (Schumacher et al. 2003; Diener 1994).

Social Desirability

To measure and control the tendency towards socially desirable behavior, we also included a social desirability scale. We assembled this scale with items from the German personality inventory FPI-R (Fahrenberg et al. 2001), for which previous research has reported satisfactory psychometric properties as well (Fahrenberg et al. 2001).

2.3.2 *Results of Study 2*

2.3.2.1 Overall Art-of-Living-Score

First, we calculated an overall art-of-living score as the mean of all subscales. An analysis of the distribution showed that the overall score in the main sample was normally distributed.

2.3.2.2 Demographic Variables

We also checked whether the demographic variables showed an effect on the overall art-of-living score. The evaluation indicated no significant effects of age, sex, family/relationship status, children, or education on art-of-living.

2.3.2.3 Research Questions 5, 6, and 7

Furthermore, we calculated various correlative relations. Table 2.6 shows the correlations between the scales and the correlation between the overall scale and the subscales (computed in the main sample, $N = 1105$). Cronbach's alphas are also presented in the diagonal of Table 2.6. Most scales showed internal consistencies greater than .70, whereas some were between .60 and .70. Only two scales (*coping* and *shaping of living conditions*) were lower and should be handled with caution. The overall art-of-living score had a consistency of .95.

Regarding the correlations it can be seen that the overall scale shows significant and high correlations (>.50) with all its subscales, which qualifies art-of-living as an overall construct. In addition, the correlations show that the sub-constructs have sufficient specificity to be of interest on their own.

Table 2.6 Means, SD, correlations and Cronbach's alpha of subscales

	OT	BA	SD	SE	SK	PC	SA	CO[a]	PA	SR	OP	SC	SL[a]	ID	Total	Mean	SD
Optimization	.69[b]															3.07	.63
Balance	.51**	.61														3.50	.66
Self-determined way of living	.60**	.53**	.77													3.56	.64
Self-efficacy	.68**	.55**	.65**	.88												3.18	.62
Self-knowledge	.55**	.52**	.68**	.60**	.72											3.67	.58
Physical care	.35**	.36**	.40**	.33**	.32**	.82										3.39	.83
Savoring	.33**	.33**	.38**	.31**	.30**	.29**	.64									3.23	.72
Coping[a]	.51**	.51**	.54**	.67**	.53**	.28**	.35**	.52								3.09	.57
Positive attitude towards life	.47**	.54**	.69**	.61**	.51**	.37**	.45**	.55**	.78							3.63	.67
Serenity	.39**	.27**	.29**	.32**	.21**	.20**	.30**	.35**	.34**	.77						2.50	.93
Openness	.37**	.41**	.51**	.52**	.39**	.32*	.21**	.48**	.48**	.28**	.70					3.49	.68
Social contact	.32**	.40**	.46**	.26**	.37**	.30**	.26**	.30**	.46**	.18**	.38**	.65				3.88	.71
Shaping of living conditions[a]	.40**	.32**	.55**	.38**	.37**	.29**	.25**	.30**	.44**	.19**	.24**	.46**	.53			3.56	.75
Integrating diff. areas of living	.49**	.35**	.47**	.37**	.30**	.37**	.50**	.34**	.39**	.37**	.23**	.29**	.35**	.63		2.62	.86
Overall art-of-living score	.75**	.69**	.84**	.81**	.71**	.55**	.55**	.73**	.80**	.80**	.64**	.56**	.57**	.60**	.95	46.36	6.45

$N = 1105$

OT optimization, *BA* balance, *SD* self-determined way of living, *SE* self-efficacy, *SK* self-knowledge, *PC* physical care, *SA* savoring, *CO* coping, *PA* positive attitude towards life, *SR* serenity, *OP* openness, *SC* social contact, *SL* shaping of living conditions, *ID* integrating different areas of living, *Total* overall Art-of-living score

** $p < .01$ (2-tailed)

[a]Caution: scale shows low reliability

[b]Diagonal elements = Cronbach's alpha

To show that our subscales provide acceptable factors for further analyses, we performed confirmatory factor analyses on basis of the items using the program Mplus (Muthén and Muthén 2009). Following the item-level factor analyses, the items were combined into parcels (i.e., small groups of items) to reduce the measurement error of items (cf. Little et al. 2002, for the pros and cons of using parcels).

The parcels were generated using the data analysis program R with an algorithm contained in the package "Psych" (Revelle 2012). The loading matrix produced by the confirmatory factor analyses is shown in Table 2.7, which also shows that all the loadings were significant. The correlations between the factors were all significant as well. The statistics assessing model fit showed an acceptable fit of the model, although the fit was not perfect: The Root Mean Square Error of Approximation (RMSEA) was .05, the fit indices were .92 for the Comparative Fit Index (CFI). Due to similarities between items we allowed 38 correlations of the item-error variables. In sum, the results of the confirmatory factor analysis justify performing studies on the level of the subscales.

Exploratory factor analyses based on the subscales resulted in a one-factor solution. The scree-test revealed a clear break after the first eigenvalue, which was 6.35 and explained 45 % of the total variance.

We also computed confirmatory factor analyses to further support this general factor model of art-of-living.

When we computed a one-factor model on the basis of the subscales, we got an RMSEA of .086, a CFI of .92, a TLI of .90, and an SRMR of .043 with highly significant loadings (cf. Table 2.8). These results show that a general factor model can be applied.

2.3.2.4 Research Questions 8 and 9

Table 2.9 contains the correlations with the scale social desirability in one column. It can be seen that even though there were a lot of significant correlations between art-of-living subscales and social desirability, there was only one correlation higher than .15 in absolute value. In sum, the analyses show that the answers on art-of-living questionnaire were hardly influenced by social desirability.

To test the hypothesis that art-of-living is positively correlated with satisfaction with life, we calculated the correlation between the overall art-of-living score and the satisfaction with life score (cf. Table 2.8). The resulting correlation of the overall scale was $r = .69$ ($p < .001$), being highly significant, which indicates that art-of-living is highly related to happiness and well-being. In matters of the relations of the subscales, each correlation was significant. The highest relation was found for a *self-determined way of living* ($r = .73$) and the lowest for *serenity* ($r = .26$).

Table 2.7 Loadings of factor analyses based on parcels

	OT	BA	SD	SE	SK	PC	SA	CO[a]	PA	SR	OP	SC	SL[a]	ID
P_ OT1	.47/.03													
P_OT2	.71/.02													
P_OT3	.73/.02													
P_ BA1		.69/.03												
P_ BA2		.52/.03												
P_SD1			.73/.02											
P_SD2			.75/.02											
P_SD3			.66/.02											
P_SE1				.80/.01										
P_SE2				.79/.01										
P_SE3				.68/.02										
P_SE4				.78/.01										
P_SE5				.71/.02										
P_SK1					.72/.02									
P_SK2					.60/.02									
P_SK3					.66/.02									
P_ PC1						.90/.02								
P_ PC2						.87/.02								
P_ SA1							.57/.03							
P_ SA2							.63/.03							
P_CO[a]1								.72/.02						
P_CO[a]2								.47/.03						
P_CO[a]3								.35/.03						

(continued)

Table 2.7 (continued)

	OT	BA	SD	SE	SK	PC	SA	CO[a]	PA	SR	OP	SC	SL[a]	ID
P_PA1									.73/ .02					
P_PA2									.82/ .01					
P_PA3									.53/ .03					
P_ SR1										.69/ .01				
P_ SR2										.91/ .02				
P_OP1											.74/ .02			
P_OP2											.47/ .03			
P_OP3											.62/ .02			
P_ SC1												.66/ .03		
P_ SC2												.62/ .03		
P_SL[a]1													.35/ .04	
P_SL[a]2													.45/ .04	
I_ID1														.57/ .03
I_ID2														.68/ .02
I_ID3														.55/ .03

Values loadings/*SD;* correlations of measurement errors were admitted according to the level of Modification Indices

[a]Caution: scale shows low reliability

OT optimization, *BA* balance, *SD* self-determined way of living, *SE* self-efficacy, *SK* self-knowledge, *PC* Physical care, *SA* savoring, *CO* coping, *PA* positive attitude towards life, *SR* serenity, *OP* openness, *SC* social contact, *SL* shaping of living conditions, *ID* integrating different areas of living, *P* paracel, *I* Item

In addition, we performed a multiple regression analysis to predict subjective well-being by all art-of-living subscales. All variables were included in the prediction equation and showed a significant contribution to the prediction, except *physical care*, *coping* and *serenity*. The remaining 11 variables resulted in $R = .78$, $R^2 = .61$, $F(11,1093) = 170{,}4$; $p < .001$. Thus it appears that well-being can be predicted very well by art-of-living, nearly all variables contribute to the prediction and more than 60 % of the variance of the criterion can be explained.

Table 2.8 Loadings of the subscales of the one-factor solution

Optimization	.73 (.02)
Balance	.68 (.02)
Self-determined way of living	.85 (.01)
Self-efficacy	.78 (.01)
Self-knowledge	.72 (.02)
Physical care	.48 (.02)
Savoring	.47 (.03)
Coping	.68 (.02)
Positive attitude towards life	.79 (.01)
Serenity	.41 (.03)
Openness	.59 (.02)
Social contact	.54 (.02)
Shaping of living conditions	.55 (.02)
Integrating different areas of living	.53 (.02)

Values in parentheses = SD

Table 2.9 Correlations of the scales with other instruments for validation

	Subjective well-being	Social desirability	Overall art-of-living score
Subjective well-being	–	.02	.69**
Overall Art-of-living score	.69**	.14**	–
Optimization	.56**	.12**	.75**
Balance	.40**	.05	.69**
Self-determined way of living	.73**	.08**	.84**
Self-efficacy	.55**	-.01	.81**
Self-knowledge	.46**	.08**	.71**
Physical care	.32**	.02	.55**
Savoring	.35**	.02	.55**
Coping	.41**	.05	.73**
Positive attitude towards life	.63**	.09**	.80**
Serenity	.26**	.36**	.51**
Openness	.34**	.09**	.64**
Social contact	.41**	.11**	.56**
Shaping of living conditions	.56**	.08**	.57**
Integrating different areas of living	.48**	.12**	.60**

*** $p < .001$; ** $p < .01$; * $p < .05$

2.3.2.5 Research Question 4: Are There Different Types of Art-of-Living?

A cluster analysis was conducted in order to find out whether there were subgroups of participants with respect to the subscales of art-of-living. All subscales were integrated. We applied the SPSS classification program *two-step-cluster*, which automatically detects the number of clusters and computes the mean values for each cluster. The results indicated a three-cluster solution. Cluster 1 contained 265 individuals (24 %), Cluster 2 contained 576 individuals (52.2 %), and Cluster 3 contained 264 individuals (24 %). The clusters can be organized in an ascending order. In Cluster 1, the participants with low scores were assorted; in Cluster 2, the participants who achieved medium scores were merged; and classified for Cluster 3 were only individuals with high values for each subscale. The results show that the profiles are parallel, and the clusters differ only with respect to the overall score of art-of-living, no qualitatively different subtypes could be found. This brings up the fact that individuals can be characterized as either low, medium, or high in art-of-living, irrespective of the kind of subscale that was in focus. This result is in line with the high correlations of the subscales and the one-dimensional factor structure on the level of the subscales.

Note that this does not mean that all individual art-of-living profiles were similar despite their general level. In fact, there was high variability among the individual profiles, but there were no common profiles leading to subtypes.

Additionally, we performed a latent class analysis, which serves a purpose similar to the cluster analysis, but uses a totally different method. In order to allow comparison with the results from the cluster analysis, we computed a latent class analysis with three latent classes. The results are shown in Fig. 2.1.

Again, the three classes can be put into an ascending order. The means of the classes for the subscales show three classes with results similar to the cluster analysis.

Therefore, we can conclude that there were no homogeneous subtypes for art-of-living, classes and clusters differed only in the general amount of art-of-living. However, the high variability among the individual profiles shows that the individual profiles differ greatly.

2.3.2.6 Research Question 2: Can Art-of-Living Be Learned?

We presented results to this research question in study 1. We now add results from study 2. In line with Schmid's (2004) and our theory of art-of-living, one would assume art-of-living can be learned. However, this assumption has important implications, namely, whether it makes sense to teach art-of-living in schools or to develop trainings to enhance art-of-living in individuals. Therefore, we wanted to verify it relying on empirical data. Clearly, this question can be answered best by using a control group design to demonstrate that teaching or training art-of-living leads to enhancement of the same. But still, to see how our sample thought about

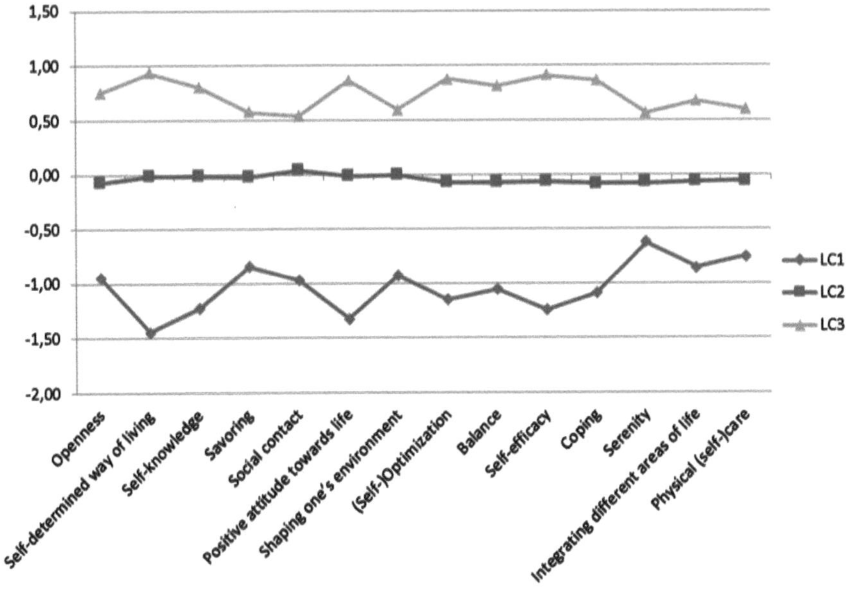

Fig. 2.1 Results of the latent class analysis, grouping the participants by their level of overall art-of-living: participants in LC1 had lower scores, participants in LC2 had medium scores and participants in LC3 had the highest scores of art-of-living

this issue, we asked our participants to evaluate the statement: "Everyone can learn how to live a full life." The frequencies of the answers were: *does not apply at all*, $n = 14$ (1.3 %); *does not apply*, $n = 42$ (3.8 %); *rather does not apply*, $n = 135$ (12.2 %); *rather does apply*, $n = 350$ (31.7 %); *applies*, $n = 408$ (36.9 %); *totally applies*, $n = 156$ (14.1 %). In sum, 82.7 % of the sample rather agreed, agreed, or totally agreed with the idea that art-of-living can be learned.

2.3.2.7 Research Question 3: Is There Only One Way to Live a Full Life?

We also presented results to this research question in study 1. We now add results from study 2. In a similar way, we wanted to know whether there is only one way to perform art-of-living. To find out how our sample thought about this issue, we asked our participants to respond to the statement: "There is only one way to live a full life." The frequencies of the answers were: *totally applies*, $n = 19$ (1.7 %); *applies*, $n = 31$ (2.8 %); *rather does apply*, $n = 53$ (4.8 %); *rather does not apply*, $n = 233$ (21.1 %); *does not apply*, $n = 377$ (34.1 %); *does not apply at all*, $n = 392$ (35.5 %). In sum, 90.7 % of the sample rather didn't agree, didn't agree, or totally disagreed, indicating that the majority did not believe that there is only one way of pursuing art-of-living.

2.4 Discussion Study 1 and 2

Our study and the resulting questionnaire represent theoretical progress in the field of art-of-living. The questionnaire comprises 14 scales and 79 corresponding items. It shows satisfactory psychometric properties and can be completed online in about 15 min. The measured art-of-living value is correlated with satisfaction with life. The independence of art-of-living from demographic variables supports our postulation that art-of-living can be achieved by different types of individuals.

The fact that there were no remarkable correlations with social desirability shows that it is unlikely that the answers in art-of-living questionnaire are determined by a need for positive self-description.

The cluster analysis shows that participants can be classified into three groups. The results indicate that participants generally achieve either high, medium, or low scores on all scales. There is no existence of different subtypes within the group with high scores in art-of-living. Although there is a lot of variability between the individual profiles, no common subtypes could be detected.

Different analyses indicate the importance of the scales *self-determined way of living, optimism*, and *self-efficacy* for the concept of art-of-living. The scales show the highest correlation with the overall score and with satisfaction with life. The evaluation of the preliminary interview had already indicated the relevance of these components. Most participants connected art-of-living mainly to *optimism*, *coping with negative events*, and a *self-determined way of living*.

2.4.1 Limitations Study 1 and 2

Some limitations of the study have to be taken into consideration.

The scales *coping* and *shaping of living conditions* showed low reliabilities; thus, they have to be interpreted with caution. As we still consider these components to be relevant to the construct of art-of-living, the scales and items have to be revised for future studies.

It has to be taken into account that the questionnaire was presented as an online version. Therefore, the sample is not fully representative of the whole population. People without computers and the internet were excluded from our study. This could be a disadvantage as elderly people were excluded, and they might be of special interest regarding questions about art-of-living. Another disadvantage is that the amounts of women and men were not equally distributed in our sample (more female participants). We assume that women are more interested in questions about art-of-living than men. As we did not establish any normed values with our sample, this unequal distribution should not be considered a serious problem.

Regarding the questions about the possibility of learning art-of-living and the number of ways to perform art-of-living, we used only one item for each question. Therefore, it could be assumed that these questions contain an implicit message about how to answer (e.g., that they invite individuals to answer in a certain way). But because our open questions in the interviews (e.g., "art-of-living is something only for people who were born as artists of living.") are free of suggesting any concrete answer, the possibility of bias because of the answer format is not probable.

With respect to the conceptualization and measurement of art-of-living, we entered a new field, and therefore, we do not believe that we reached a final point. Instead, we view our concept and our questionnaire as the first steps in this direction.

2.4.2 *Outlook Study 1 and 2*

We tried to transfer the concept of art-of-living, which has a long tradition in philosophy, to psychological research. We pursued this idea from the 2003 special issue in the Journal of Happiness Studies (Veenhoven 2003a, b). Firstly we have conducted a study on the philosophical background by Wilhelm Schmid (2004). Now we began our empirical study by interviewing a sample of participants about their understanding of basic concepts of art-of-living. Based on this data and the philosophical background, we further elaborated our concept of art-of-living and developed a questionnaire to get an empirical foundation for its measurement. The project was successful in that we presented an instrument with satisfactory statistical properties. The overall internal consistency was quite high (which was not surprising because of the number of items), but also most of the subscales showed sufficient consistency. In addition, we demonstrated that subjective well-being could be predicted very well by art-of-living because the correlation between the overall art-of-living scale and subjective well-being was .69, the multiple correlation was .78, and the R^2 value was .61. This could be interpreted that high art-of living values can lead to high well-being. Moreover, we demonstrated that our art-of-living measure was only minimally influenced by social desirability. Regarding the factorial structure, analyses on the scale level showed that it makes sense to view art-of-living as an overall construct, whereas more detailed analyses of the items showed that it makes sense to have a look at the subscales. The analyses of the latent classes and the cluster analyses led to similar results but from different methodological perspectives. The results showed that there were not different subgroups with homogeneous profiles but rather with different general levels. The individual profiles were rather different but no common profiles were found. This is in line with the view (and also corresponding to Schmid) that there are many different ways to perform art-of-living.

We do not assume that our concept will be the final answer to the question how art-of-living can be conceptualized and measured. We rather believe that this is a first but important step in supporting the development of the psychological study of art-of-living on an empirical basis. Future studies might add other constructs (e.g., personality, wisdom), which might be important or might further sharpen the contours of the concept and its measurement.

Regarding the question whether art-of-living can be learned, we, along with Schmid and our sample, agree. The instrument that was introduced in this chapter could be used to evaluate interventions that try to enhance art-of-living. The ways in which this can be done are numerous (see e.g., studies by Fordyce 1977, 1983; Sin and Lyubomirsky 2009; Seligman et al. 2006). Future studies might evaluate such interventions using our questionnaire to measure art-of-living.

2.5 Study 3

2.5.1 Art-of-Living Questionnaire: Revised Edition

In the first stage of the development of the questionnaire for art-of-living the theoretical ground was mainly Schmid's (2004) philosophical considerations. But as described in chapter one also the rapidly growing knowledge of positive psychology has to be integrated. Therefore a refinement of the first conception seems to be rational. There are empirical and theoretical considerations, because the instrument development is an ongoing process we want to optimize the instrument from the perspective of test-quality criteria, to reach better homogeneity measures but also a better theoretical representation of the core concept. Although we see *meaning* as a central component of art-of-living, until now *meaning* was only a part of *self-determined way of living*. Therefore we decided to split off *meaning* from *self-determined way of living*. From the study of humanistic literature, e.g. Maslow (1968), Rogers (1961), we believe that a tendency to self-actualization to strive for growth and personal development would be an important component that was neglected in the first concept. A third component we missed in our primary approach was reflection. Because in our personal research history we investigated learning, education and self-regulation there it become apparent that metacognition is important for learning and generally enhancing one's quality of life. Because life-long learning is important one has to think about what one has done, to evaluate one's behavior in order to find out what was good and what not and as consequence to change behavior if necessary. Note however, that reflection is a complicated topic. Well-known are the pitfalls of rumination, cf. Nolen-Hoeksema (2004) where this kind of reflection does not lead to any positive consequences. Rumination involves repeating of negative thoughts, which could lead to depression. Also ineffective is reflection without action, e.g. in case of procrastinating: having goals without doing very much to reach them (Steel, 2007). Other constructs we thought about to include to art-of-living was for example humor. But we were not sure about its status in the hierarchy. We find it very important to have humor, it helps in

Table 2.10 New scales with sample items

Scale	Sample item
Reflection	"I try to analyze and to evaluate my behavior in retrospect"
Self-actualization	"I seek to actualize my potential"
Meaning	"I work towards the achievement of my personal objectives"

many life situations (Ruch 1998). But compared to other constructs it seems to be on a hierarchical lower level, e.g. as special coping strategy. Also an important topic is transcendence, e.g. to believe in god or a higher instance. Transcendence is also contained in the Strength and Virtues catalog of Peterson and Seligman (2004). But from our perspective it is a special strategy belonging to the category of *meaning* and therefore it is also can be considered as construct on a different level.

In sum, from a theoretical perspective we additionally include *self-actualization, meaning* and *reflection* from an empirical test criteria perspective we try to enhance especially *shaping of living conditions* and *coping.*

Now we turn to the empirical revision. Both the scales and items included in the art-of-living questionnaire were revised. We present a brief overview over the changes and improvements.

Preparatory to another study (Sample: N = 150, 93 % university students, mean age 24.5, SD = 4.7) three scales were added (see Table 2.10). Moreover, further items were added to nearly all of the scales. Some specific scales like *coping* or *shaping of living conditions* were changed virtually completely. The core components of the scale *self-determined way of living* were divided into two separate scales as described above, one *meaning* and the other one with the same label as before: *self-determined way of living.*

2.5.1.1 Was the Revision's Outcome Satisfactory?

While analyzing the questionnaire it became evident that consistencies improved in virtually all categories. The accuracy of measurement improved particularly for *balance, coping, shaping of living conditions, enjoyment, positive attitude towards life itself, social life* and *self-knowledge,* see Table 2.11.

The revision of the art-of-living questionnaire could be viewed as successful. It is on a theoretical basis improved and the consistencies for the subscales now are sufficient.

2.6 Study 4

Janina Linten, Bettina Schumacher

Table 2.11 The scales' reliabilities in comparison between the main study and the collegiate study

Scales	Item count	α Main study	α Collegiate study
Balance	6	.61	.69
Coping	7	.52	.74
Serenity	6	.77	.79
Savoring	8	.64	.75
Shaping of living conditions	5	.53	.82
Physical care	6	.82	.86
Openness	7	.70	.68
Optimization	7	.69	.73
Positive attitude towards life	10	.78	.85
Reflection	9	–	.79
Self-actualization	8	–	.82
Self-knowledge	11	.72	.86
Self-determined way of living	7	.77	.72
Self-efficacy	7	.88	.80
Meaning	10	–	.86
Social contact	9	.65	.81
Integrating different areas of living	5	.63	.55
Art-of-living total (items)	78/127	.95	.96
Art-of-living total (scales)	14/17	.86	.91

2.6.1 A Shortened Form of the Art-of-Living Questionnaire

The revised version of the art-of-living questionnaire fulfills the criterion for sufficient internal consistencies for the subscales. It allows a differentiated diagnosis of the individual status for art-of-living. But the questionnaire is rather lengthy. Compared to the VIA it consists of the half number of items, but for many contexts it needs a too long time to answer all the questions. Therefore, we want to develop a shortened version which could be applied in a multitude of situations. In a first trial, we applied an empirical approach in that we are aiming to identify the items with the highest factor loading and thereby to generate a valid, reliable and economical abbreviated version of the art-of-living-questionnaire the data from a 2015 online study (N = 636) was evaluated in a parallel analysis. The resulting 14-factor-model was subjected to an exploratory factor analysis with oblique rotation (*Oblimin*). The empirical χ^2-value was 6976.43 ($p < .05$), the TLI (Tucker-Lewis-Index) amounted to .875, RMSEA (Root Mean Square Error Approximation) was .033 and the BIC (Bayesian Information Criterion) was −33,317.03.

As a consequence both items with low factor loading (<.3) and those that could not be identified as a component of any factor were excluded. Afterwards the resulting data was subjected to a parallel analysis once more.

This process was repeated until the TLI reached a sound value of .988. The model was reduced to a 10-factor-model comprising 30 items. All factor loadings exceeded .50 while the empirical χ^2-value amounted to 72.8 ($p < .1$). RMSEA was .021 and Cronbach's alpha for the entire model was .90, whereas Cronbach's alpha for each of the scales yielded between .77 and .88.

The final abridged edition consisted of 9 scales taken from the original version as well as an additional scale *goal-orientation,* which has its origin in the *meaningfulness*-scale. The scales were measured by three items each. The abbreviated edition was then validated again with a sample of students (N = 241; mean age = 25.22; SD = 4.8; 55.6 % female). The resulting reliabilities are between .74 and .89. In addition, participants also stated their satisfaction with life (SWLS). It could be shown that art-of-living predicted SWLS with R = . 65 $R^2 = .42$, F (1239) = 149.5, $p = < .001$.

Even though the fit indices are quite well, we are not fully satisfied with this short form and try to enhance it.

2.7 Overall Discussion

Designing the art-of-living-questionnaire began with the goal to merge the various theoretical and philosophical aspects and constructs into one empirically validated instrument producing precise and reliable measurements. In the process of different tests and studies including qualitative and quantitative data a valid, reliable questionnaire designed to have a psychological measure for art-of-living was created.

References

Bortz, J., & Döring, N. (2006). *Forschungsmethoden und Evaluation für Human- und Sozialwissenschaftler* (4th ed.). Heidelberg: Springer.

Diener, E. (1994). Assessing subjective well-being: Progress and opportunities. *Social Indicators Research, 31*, 103–157.

Diener, E., Emmons, R. A., Larsen, R. J., & Griffin, S. (1985). The satisfaction with life scale. *Journal of Personality Assessment, 49*(1), 71–75.

Fahrenberg, J., Hampel, R., & Selg, H. (2001). Das Freiburger Persönlichkeitsinventar FPI-*R* (7. überarbeitete und neu normierte ed.) [The Freiburg Personality Inventory FPI-R] . Göttigen: Hogrefe.

Fordyce, M. W. (1977). Development of a program to increase personal happiness. *Journal of Counseling Psychology, 24*, 511–521.

Fordyce, M. W. (1983). A program to increase happiness: Further studies. *Journal of Counseling Psychology, 30*, 483–498.

Hinz, A., Schumacher, J., Albani, C., Schmid, G., & Brähler, E. (2006). Bevölkerungsrepräsentative Normierung der Skala zur Allgemeinen Selbstwirksamkeitserwartung [A representative normalization of the scale *general self-efficacy*]. *Diagnostica, 52*(1), 26–32.

Little, T. D., Cunningham, W. A., Shahar, G., & Widaman, K. F. (2002). To parcel or not to parcel: Exploring the question, weighing the merits. *Structural Equation Modeling, 9*(2), 151–173.

Maslow, A. H. (1968). *Toward a psychology of being* (2nd ed.). New York: Van Nostrand.
Muthén, B., & Muthén, B. O. (2009). *Statistical analysis with latent variables*. New York: Wiley.
Nolen-Hoeksema, S. (2004). The response styles theory. In C. Papageorgiou & A. Wells (Eds.), *Depressiv rumination: Nature, theory, and treatment* (pp. 107–124). Chichester, UK: Wiley.
Peterson, C., & Seligman, M. E. (2004). *Character strengths and virtues: A handbook and classification*. Oxford: Oxford University Press.
Revelle, W. (2012). Procedures for psychological, psychometric, and personality research. Retrieved February 16, 2012, from http://cran.r-project.org/web/packages/psych/psych.pdf.
Rogers, C. R. (1961). *On becoming a person: A therapist's viwe of psychotherapy*. Boston: Houghton Mifflin.
Ruch, W. (Ed.). (1998). *The sense of humor: Explorations of a personality characteristic* (Vol. 3). Berlin: Walter de Gruyter.
Schmid, W. (2004). *To be friends with ourselves—About the art of living with oneself*. Berlin: Suhrkamp Publishers.
Schumacher, J., Klaiberg, A., & Brähler, E. (Eds.). (2003). *Diagnostische Verfahren zu Lebensqualität und Wohlbefinden*. Göttingen: Hogrefe.
Seligman, M. E. P., Rashid, T., & Parks, A. C. (2006). Positive psychotherapy. *American Psychologist, 61*, 774–788.
Sin, N. L., & Lyubomirsky, S. (2009). Enhancing well-being and alleviating depressive symptoms with positive psychology interventions: A practice-friendly meta-analysis. *Journal of Clinical Psychology, 65*, 467–487.
Steel, P. (2007). The nature of procrastination: A meta-analytic and theoretical review of quintessential self-regulatory failure. *Psychological Bulletin, 133*(1), 65.
Veenhoven, R. (2003a). Notions of art-of-living. Introduction to this special issue. *Journal of Happiness Studies, 4*, 345–349.
Veenhoven, R. (2003b). Arts-of-living. *Journal of Happiness Studies, 4*, 373–384.

Chapter 3
Validation Studies for Art-of-Living

3.1 Relationships of Art-of-Living to Different Constructs of Well-Being

Bernhard Schmitz, Katharina Treichel, Bettina Schumacher, Alice Lautz and Janina Linten

3.1.1 Introduction

In the introduction (Chap. 1) we have described main constructs of well-being. Within our approach we regard well-being as a criterion for a good life which can be enhanced by using art-of-living strategies. We have already introduced subjective well-being, psychological well-being and eudaimonic well-being and will analyze the relationship of art-of-living and these constructs. Because the enhancement of well-being and of art-of-living are the topics of this book we want to discuss main constructs of well-being research. Therefore, we not only include the constructs mentioned above in our validation approach, but also two other concepts of well-being, namely authentic happiness (AHI) and subjective happiness (SHS). Additionally, in many studies a measure of depression is included to well-being, and the meta-analysis from Sin and Lyubomirsky (2009) reports statistics not only for well-being but also to depression.

3.1.1.1 Concept of Authentic Happiness (AHI)

The concept of authentic happiness goes back to Seligman et al. (2005). The idea was to measure well-being in a similar way to depression, e.g. CES-D (Center for Epidemiological Studies-Depression, Radloff 1977). Because the authors missed an

B. Schmitz, *Art-of-Living*, Social Indicators Research Series 63,
DOI 10.1007/978-3-319-45324-8_3

instrument including the three orientations to happiness, positive emotion, engagement and meaning, they developed the SHI (Steen happiness index). The intention was that the SHI should capture changes in happiness in a similar way the SES-D allows for changes in depressive symptoms. Empirical tests of the SHI yielded a better bell-shaped distribution than similar measures. The actual form of this instrument is the AHI (authentic happiness inventory).

3.1.1.2 Subjective Happiness Scale (SHS)

Lyubomirsky and Lepper (1999) developed this scale for measuring global subjective happiness. Instead of asking for positive and negative affect, the subjects should report whether they felt like a happy or an unhappy person. Another aspect asked for was the happiness in comparison to other people.

3.1.1.3 Depression

As part of the concept of *learned helplessness* Seligman (1995) designed a model of depression. Thus, possible depressive symptoms are inter alia persistent or repetitive feelings of sadness, exhaustion and listlessness, passivity, loss of weight and libido, social withdrawal and suicidal thoughts. Sin and Lyubomirsky (2009) showed in their meta-analysis, that positive interventions both reduce depressive symptoms and boost well-being effectively. From the Positive Psychology research resulted a kind of psychotherapeutic treatment (*positive therapy*) to encounter depression, which not only aims on reducing negative symptoms but also building positive emotions. Thus, well-being can be described as pendant to depression.

In the following we look at the relationships between different well-being measures as well as depression and art-of-living total scale and subscales.

We make the following assumptions. First art-of-living total scale is related to all measures of well-being. We argue that art-of-living is a holistic and integrative construct of strategies and attitudes towards leading a good life. Therefore art-of-living should be related to different outcome measures of leading a good life which is well-being.

In the same way we assume that all art-of-living subcomponents are aspects of leading a good life, they should result in well-being. Clearly this does not hold for all the subscales of psychological well-being because they measure specific aspects of well-being.

The relationship between total art-of-living and the general well-being measures SWLS and AHI and SHS will be higher than between art-of-living and EWB because EWB focuses more on meaning aspects.

Second, on the level of subconstructs similar constructs of art-of-living and psychological well-being will be correlated, e.g. *meaning* (art-of-living) will be related to meaning (psychological well-being) *social contact* (art-of-living) will be related to relationships (psychological well-being) and *shaping of living conditions* (art-of-living) will be related to environment (psychological well-being).

Thirdly, total art-of-living will be strongly related to autonomy (psychological well-being) because *self-determined way of living* and therefore autonomy is a main aspect of art-of-living.

Fourthly, according to our understanding of depression as counterpart to well-being, we expect negative correlations between depression and art of living total as well as art-of-living subscales.

3.1.2 Method

3.1.2.1 Sample

Sample 1 for *subjective happiness* and *satisfaction with life* recorded by Schumacher (2015), included 636 participants with a stake of 81.60 % females. The mean age amounted to 27.61 years (*SD* = 10.64). 47 % participants were single, 31 % in a relationship and 16 % married. Most participants had an A level certificate (65 %), or completed studies (23 %) respectively were an active student (62 %).

Sample 2 for *authentic happiness* recorded by Lautz (2013), included 242 participants of which 76 % were female. The mean age was 29.31 years (*SD* = 10.39). Most participants were unmarried (65 %). Most participants had an A level certificate (48 %), or completed studies (33 %) respectively were an active student (41 %).

Sample 3 for *psychological well-being* comprised 150 participants. They were students at an university. There is no more information about the sample.

Sample 4 for *eudaimonic well-being*, collected by Treichel (2015) comprised 201 participants respectively of which 71.6 % were female with a mean ages of 32 (*SD* = 13.70) years. Almost one third in each case was in a relationship (33 %) or married (35 %). Most of participants had an A level certificate (40 %), or completed studies (27 %).

3.1.2.2 Instruments

In addition to the revised questionnaire of art-of-living (Chap. 2) we applied the following instruments.

Authentic Happiness Inventory (AHI)

For measuring happiness according to Seligman we used the AHI which contains 24 items (Seligman et al. 2005). Each item consists of five statements, which range from negative to positive and are provided with letters from A to E. Participants choose one of them to specify their well-being with respect to the last week. An example item is: (A) *I am unhappy with myself.* (B) *I am neither happy nor unhappy with myself- I am neutral.* (C) *I am happy with myself.* (D) *I am very happy with myself.* (E) *I could not be happier with myself.* Schiffrin and Nelson (2010) reported Cronbach's α of .92. This value was replicated in the present study (α = .93).

Subjective Happiness Scale (SHS)

Lyubomirsky and Lepper (1999) developed this scale for measuring global subjective happiness. One example item is: *In general, I consider myself* (1) *not a very happy person*... or (7) *a very happy person.* Another aspect is the happiness in comparison to peers, for example: *Compared to most of my peers, I consider myself* (1) *less happy*... or (7) *more happy*. The questionnaire contains four items with this 7-pointed Likert scale. The authors report internal consistency (Cronbach's α) from .79 to .94 in 14 different samples. In the present study resulted .81.

Questionnaire for Psychological Wellbeing (PWB)

The self-report questionnaire of Ryff and Keyes (1995) measures the psychological well-being with 18 items belonging to six subscales: environment (*In general, I feel I am in charge of the situation in which I live*), self-growth (*I think that it is important to have new experiences that challenge how you think about yourself and the world*), relationships (*People would describe me as a giving person, willing to share my time with others*), meaning (*Some people wander aimlessly through life, but I am not one of them*), self-acceptance (*I like most aspects of my personality*), and autonomy (*I have confidence in my opinions, even if contrary to the general consensus*). The self-evaluation is specified by a 6-pointed Likert scale ranging from *strong disagreement* to *strong agreement*. In the study of Ryff and Keyes Cronbach's α is .60, we found α = .78.

Questionnaire for Eudaimonic Well-Being (EWB)

Waterman et al. (2010) conceptualized this questionnaire to measure eudaimonic well-being, cf. Chap. 1. It contains the following scales: *self-discovery, perceived development of one's best potentials, a sense of purpose and meaning in life, investment of significant effort in pursuit of excellence, intense involvement in activities,* and *enjoyment of activities as personally expressive*. This instrument consists of 21 items which are answered with a 5-pointed Likert scale ranging from *strongly disagree* to *strongly agree*. An example items is: *I believe I have discovered who I really am.* Cronbach's α is .86.

Beck-Depression-Inventory (BDI)

The self-assessment tool goes back to Beck et al. (1961) and captures the extent of typical depressive symptoms, for example sadness, feeling of guilt, and social withdrawal. The subject's consent to the 21 items is specified by a 4-pointed Likert-scale ranging from *never* to *always*. An example item is (0) *I don't have any feelings of guilt,* (1) *I have often feelings of guilt,* (2) *I almost always have feelings of guilt,* (3) *I always have feelings of guilt.* The internal consistency (Cronbach's α) showed to be between .73 and .95 (Beck et al. 1996). In the present study resulted .90.

3.1.3 Results

We will present our results with respect to our assumptions. First, we look at the relationships of total art-of-living and well-being and depression, s. Table 3.1. First, looking at line one, it should be noted that the relationships between art-of-living overall and the well-being constructs SWLS, SHS and AHI are strong, $\geq .59$, and significant. The relationships for art-of-living overall and psychological well-being (PWB; $\geq .33$) and eudaimonic well-being (EWB; .38), and depression (BDI; −.57) are medium to strong and significant. Therefore our assumption holds. Furthermore all art-of-living subscales correlate significantly with the general well-being measures SWLS, AHI, SHS, EWB and BDI (inversely) with the only exception of reflection.

Also, as expected, the correlation between art-of-living and SWLS, AHI, SHS is higher than that of art-of-living with eudaimonic well-being.

On the level of corresponding subconstructs *meaning* (art-of-living) with meaning (psychological well-being) the correlation is with .39 significant and the highest in the meaning column of psychological well-being. *Social contact* (art-of-living) and relationships (psychological well-being) is .70 and again the highest correlation in the relationship column, whereas environment (psychological well-being) is .46 and there is only one correlation in the shaping of living conditions line (art-of-living) which is marginally higher.

Also as expected, the correlation between total art-of-living and autonomy (psychological well-being) is very high, in line with the concept of art-of-living as *self-determined way of living*.

Other results were: among the subconstructs of art-of-living *meaning* shows high correlations with SWLS, SHS, AHI and most of PWB. *Reflection* shows low and nonsignificant correlations with SWLS and AHI, but it shows relationships to SHS, PWB's self-growth as well as *meaning*, and EWB.

The relationships of *serenity* with well-being measures are rather low but consistent across measures. It can be seen that EWB has significant correlations with all subconstructs of art-of-living although they are low or medium. *Self-actualization* correlates with self-growth to .48 which is the highest correlation of the PWB self-growth column. Interestingly, self-acceptance shows clear relationships with

Table 3.1 Correlations of art-of-living with well-being and depression

	SWLS[a]	AHI[b]	SHS[a]	PWB[c]						EWB[d]	BDI[b]
				Environment	Self-growth	Relationships	Meaning	Self-acceptance	Autonomy		
Art-of-living total	.59***	.72***	.62***	.67***	.40***	.52***	.33***	.66***	.86***	.38***	−.57***
Balance	.28***	.46***	.38***	.34***	.18*	.33***	.16*	.45***	.30***	.33***	−.37***
Coping	.28***	.38***	.38***	.49***	.24**	.35***	.14	.42***	.31***	.27***	−.30***
Serenity	.28***	.28***	.42***	.29***	.09	.24**	.03	.27***	.11	.21**	−.36***
Savoring	.43***	.51***	.52***	.32***	.07	.29***	.01	.55***	.19*	.29***	−.45***
Self-determined way of living	.45***	.54***	.42***	.58***	.42***	.32***	.32***	.42***	.53***	.36***	−.48***
Meaning	.70***	.72***	.64***	.53***	.42***	.42***	.39***	.61***	.28***	.35***	−.56***
Social contact	.42***	.26***	.39***	.51***	.27***	.70***	.35***	.43***	.16*	.26***	−.19**
Self-efficacy	.45***	.59***	.53***	.53***	.28***	.32***	.19*	.47***	.36***	.39***	−.48***
Shaping of living conditions	.47***	.41***	.37***	.46***	.42***	.43***	.35***	.43***	.28***	.26***	−.32***
Physical care	.31***	.42***	.26***	.42***	.06	.47***	.13	.47***	.03	.28***	−.35***
Openness	.22***	.42***	.35***	.34***	.38***	.28***	.17*	.28***	.34***	.20**	−.37***
Integrating different areas of life	.42***	.48***	.35***	.60***	.11	.53***	.26**	.53***	.14	.27***	−.46***
Optimization	.51***	.60***	.42***	.67***	.27***	.50***	.35***	.50***	.36***	.41***	−.52***
Positive attitude towards life	.59***	.66***	.70***	.42***	.21**	.58***	.13	.58***	.07	.34***	−.32***
Reflection	−.06	.05	−.12**	.09	.37***	.01	.18*	.01	.14	.23***	.06
Self-actualization	.47***	.57***	.41***	.55***	.48***	.44***	.38***	.44***	.38***	.27***	−.45***
Self-knowledge	.40***	.55***	.40***	.45***	.21**	.45***	.23**	.45***	.38***	.40***	−.44***

SWLS Satisfaction with Life Scale, *AHI* Authentic Happiness Inventory, *SHS* Subjective Happiness Scale, *PWB* Psychological Well-being, *EWB* Eudemonic Well-being, *BDI* Beck-Depression-Inventory

[a] Schumacher (2015), $N = 636$; [b] Lautz (2013), $N = 242$; [c] Student Sample, $N = 150$; [d] Treichel (2015), $N = 201$

* $p < .05$; ** $p < .01$; *** $p < .001$

most of art-of-living scales, although art-of-living does not explicitly measure self-acceptance.

Furthermore, as expected, the relationship of art-of-living and depression (BDI) goes into the opposite direction: The art-of-living total score as well as the subscales except *reflection* show significant negative relationships with BDI total score. The strongest relationships regarding to the art-of-living subscales revealed for *meaning* (-.56), *optimization* (-.52), *self-determined way of living* (-.48), and *self-efficacy* (-.48). The latter three art-of-living components in particular emphasize the individual responsibility to make one's own life. That's in line with Seligman's (1995) concept of learned helplessness, in which depressive symptoms are viewed as result of experienced or adopted action inability.

In sum, as expected since art-of-living is conceptualized as ways to leading a good life, the results show that art-of-living has high and meaningful relationships to different measures of well-being as criteria for leading a good life. The relationships to depression are also significant, but negative. Note that total art-of-living and almost all the subscales correlate with all SWLS, AHI, SHS, EWB, and BDI, that means, it makes sense to include all these aspects in art-of-living, because they were all related to the different conceptualizations of well-being.

3.2 Validation: Key Constructs in Positive Psychology—Relationships Between the Art-of-Living and Flourishing

Nicole Klimek, Janina Linten, Bernhard Schmitz

3.2.1 Introduction

In Chap. 1 an overview of the various ways of leading a good life as well as their results was provided. Flourishing was part of the results of leading a good life described in Chap. 1. Therefore art-of-living as strategies and attitudes towards leading a good life should correlate with various measures of flourishing. We also assume that all subconstructs of art-of-living should be related to flourishing.

3.2.1.1 Research Objectives

It was our goal to compare the aforementioned concepts for measuring flourishing based on Hone et al. (2014; see Table 3.2) for validating the art-of-living

Table 3.2 Correlations between different measures of flourishing from Hone et al. (2014) and own study

	Keyes	Huppert et al.	Diener et al.
Results from Hone et al. (2014)[a]			
Huppert and So	.54*		
Diener et al.	.52*	.48*	
Seligman et al.	.62*	.53*	.59*
Results from our own study[b]			
Huppert et al.	.79*		
Diener et al.	.67*	.75*	
Seligman et al.	.73*	.83*	.77*

* $p < .05$. For better comparability we adjusted the significance level of our study to those of Hone et al. (2014)

[a] $N = 10{,}009$, [b] $N = 202$

questionnaire. Flourishing is regarded as the desired outcome which can be achieved with a high score in the art-of-living.

3.2.2 *Method*

3.2.2.1 Sample

The sample for flourishing comprised 202 participants respectively of which 71.3 % were female with a mean age of 38 ($SD = 15.9$) years. Almost one third in each case were single (30 %), in a relationship (29 %) or married (33 %). Most of participants had an A level certificate (36 %), or completed studies (36 %).

3.2.2.2 Instruments

Art-of-Living

The revised art-of-living-questionnaire, see Sect. 2.5 was used.

Flourishing

Table 3.3 provides a comparative overview and gives information about the authors, Cronbach's α, number of items, and scaling, and it provides an example item for each instrument. The following authors developed measures of flourishing: Seligman: PERMA-P, Keyes: Mental health continuum, Huppert & So: European Social Survey (ESS) and Diener et al.: Flourishing Scale (FS).

Table 3.3 Comparative overview of the flourishing-questionnaires

Name	Author	α	Items	Content	Scaling	Example Item
PERMA-profilers (PERMA-P)	Seligman (2011)	92	5	Based on the five elements of PERMA	11-pointed Likert-scale (*never/ always; not at all/ completely*)	Success: *How often do you feel like you have made progress with regard to your goals?*
Flourishing scale (FS)	Diener et al. (2010)	87	8	E.g. competence, meaning, optimism, self-acceptance	7-pointed Likert-scale (*strongly agree/ strongly disagree*)	Social contribution: *I actively contribute to other people's happiness and well-being*
European Social Survey (ESS)	Huppert and So (2013)	83	10	Competence, emotional stability, optimism, meaning Commitment, resilience, positive emotions, self-esteem, positive relationships, vitality	5-pointed Likert-scale (*strongly agree/ strongly disagree*) 4-pointed Likert scale (frequency of experience)	Positive relationships: *there are people in my life who are genuinely interested in a social relationship with me*
Mental Health Continuum Short Form (MHC-SF)	Keyes (2002)	89	4	Three components of well-being (emotional, social, psychological well-being	Frequency of experience during the previous month (e.g. once or twice, once a week, almost daily, daily)	Psych. well-being: *how often did you feel challenged to mature and become a better person over the events of the last month?*

Note Cronbach's α calculated in this study (Klimek 2015)

Seligman's PERMA-Profiler

For improved operationalization of flourishing Seligman (2011) developed the PERMA-profiler, which is designed to measure the five elements of well-being *positive emotions, engagement, positive relationships, meaning,* and *accomplishments.* For more information see Hone et al. (2014).

Keyes Mental Health Continuum

For the first time the term "flourishing"—in its current meaning—was used by Corey Keyes in 2002. His questionnaire already contains the essential aspects the PERMA-profiler comprises. However it also includes further scales like autonomy or social acceptance. According to Keyes' approach a high level of emotional, psychological and social well-being is required, hence it is measured in the Mental Health Continuum Short Form (MHC-SF; Keyes 2002). According to his terminology hedonistic symptoms and a positive functioning have to be evident in order to classify as flourishing (Hone et al. 2014).

Huppert & So (European Social Survey)

Huppert and So (2013, p. 838) define flourishing as a combination of feeling positive and effective functioning. Their instrument measures 10 positive attributes (see Table 3.3) comprising both eudemonistical and hedonistic aspects of well-being (Hone et al. 2014). They developed their instrument as a part of the European Social Survey (ESS).

Diener et al. Flourishing Scale

Diener et al. devised a flourishing scale in order to measure the psychological functioning complementary to the other aspects of psychological well-being (Hone et al. 2014). Based on universal psychological needs this scale combines them with other theories of well-being (Diener et al. 2010). It merges various dimensions of well-being like optimism and commitment, which are important for positive functioning (self-acceptance, meaning) according to Ryff (1989) and Ryan and Deci (2001), into a single scale.

3.2.3 Results

The analyses of the relationships between the art-of-living and the flourishing-instruments (s. Table 3.4) revealed correlations of .61 to Keyes MHC-SF flourishing scale, .75 to Huppert et al. flourishing scale, .72 to Diener et al. flourishing scale and .76 to the Seligman et al. PERMA-Profiler. That means they are all of similar amount and all >.60 so that art-of-living and flourishing show strong relationships independent of the measurement instrument, where the Keyes instrument shows slightly lower relationships. The scales *positive attitude towards life* and *meaning* show particularly high correlations to flourishing which can be explained with the partial similarity with regard to the contents between the questionnaires. Flourishing instruments also measure aspects of meaning and commitment. These elements show a connection with a generally positive attitude towards life. Interestingly, all components of art-of-living with the exception of *reflection* yield significant correlations to all flourishing variables. That seems to

Table 3.4 Correlations between the art-of-living scales and the flourishing-questionnaires

	Keyes	Huppert et al.	Diener et al.	Seligman et al.
Art-of-living total	.61***	.75***	.72***	.76***
Balance	.33***	.45***	.44***	.45***
Coping	.38***	.45***	.34***	.46***
Serenity	.31***	.44***	.27***	.29***
Savoring	.41***	.52***	.36***	.44***
Self-determined way of living	.43***	.57***	.56***	.61***
Meaning	.64***	.72***	.72***	.76***
Social contact	.44***	.51***	.63***	.63***
Self-efficacy	.51***	.66***	.57***	.58***
Shaping of living conditions	.40***	.43***	.50***	.53***
Physical care	.39***	.45***	.52***	.48***
Integrating different areas of living	.29***	.38***	.33***	.42***
Openness	.31***	.44***	.38***	.37***
Optimization	.51***	.58***	.61***	.65***
Positive attitude towards life	.61***	.78***	.68***	.75***
Reflection	−.03	−.05	.06	.02
Self-actualization	.49***	.56***	.60***	.61***
Self-knowledge	.39***	.53***	.54***	.51***

$N = 202$
*** $p < .001$

underline the usefulness to include all these components within the concept of art-of-living. Furthermore, it became evident that the inter-correlations of the various flourishing-instruments are continuously higher than Hone et al. (2014) stated (see Table 3.3).

3.2.4 Discussion

In summary, the assumptions that art-of-living is highly related to flourishing could be confirmed and the art-of-living questionnaire was validated further. In this context the structure of the correlation matrix is showing significant correlations of all subconstructs (exception *reflection*) and higher correlations to *meaning* and *positive attitude towards life* can be regarded as reasonable. As expected, the inter-correlations between the flourishing-instruments were high, showing that the differences between these instruments were not very large.

3.3 Relationship of Art-of-Living with Personality (Big Five), Anxiety, Emotional Intelligence, and Mindfulness

Alice Lautz

3.3.1 *Introduction*

The chapter at hand focuses on important constructs in personality research and their respective correlations with the art-of-living. In personality research during the last decades the five factor model of personality is well established to measure important aspects of personality (John and Srivastava 1999; McCrae and Costa 1999). Following Goldberg (1981) these factors were labelled as the *Big Five*. We want to perform analyses regarding two questions: the relationships between Big Five and the art-of-living and the incremental validity of art-of-living with respect to the Big Five in predicting well-being.

The philosopher Schmid (2004) described in his philosophical introduction to art-of-living that feelings of anxiety could lead to a confrontation with these feelings and to an intensification and an enrichment of life. We wanted to study the relationship between anxiety and art-of-living. Whereas Schmid considers that there could be a positive correlation we hypothesize a negative correlation.

Other constructs which we studied are emotional intelligence and mindfulness. Schmid (2004, S. 264) emphasizes, that emotions are indispensable for a fulfilled life. He describes three stages of dealing with emotions. First, one has to understand and interpret the quality of own emotions in an adequate manner. Second, one has to decide whether to reinforce or mitigate this emotions' quantity and third, one has to find differentiated expressions that meet the emotions' variety. This three stages of handling emotions coincide in many parts with Rindermann's (2009) psychological concept of emotional competence.

Schmid (2004) conceptualizes mindfulness (he uses the term "self-awareness", p. 79) as targeted alignment of the physical, psychological and mentally attention on something or somebody in the everyday life. Thus, mindfulness is a "source of life" (p. 80), which is available to everyone. He differentiates between inwardly and outwardly mindfulness, which are to equilibrate. The method of mindfulness already has arrived in psychological research and therapy (in behavioral therapy, see e.g. Hayes et al. 2004; Kabat-Zinn 2003 for psychoanalytic therapy see e.g. Huppertz 2003; Heidenreich and Michalak 2006), so the positive effects of mindfulness on life quality are well known.

Because emotional intelligence and mindfulness are implicit parts of art-of-living without being directly included in the questionnaire we expect significant moderate correlations.

3.3.2 Method

3.3.2.1 Sample

The sample for Big Five (N = 242; Lautz 2013) is described more in detail in Sect. 3.1.2.1.

The data for anxiety, emotional intelligence and mindfulness stem from the study of Schröder and König (2014). 178 subjects participated in the study, thereof 33.70 % males (5.10 % didn't specify their sex). The mean age was 30 years (SD = 10.70).

3.3.2.2 Instruments

For the relationships with the Big Five we applied the revised art-of-living-questionnaire, for the other analyses the original version (Schmitz and Schmidt 2014; see Chap. 2). In addition, the following instruments were used:

Big Five Inventory-Short Version (BFI-10)

In the original version the NEO-PI-R contains 240 (Costa and McCrae 1992a, b), The Big Five Inventory's abridged version with ten items (two per scale) was used for the correlational study. Rammstedt and John (2007) developed and validated this questionnaire. This economical abridged version is regarded as sufficiently reliable and valid (Rammstedt and John 2007). The factors are *extraversion*, *neuroticism*, *agreeableness*, *openness* and *conscientiousness* with Cronbach's α = .81, .77, .59, .70 and .69. In our study (N = 242) resulted α = .76, .67, .74, and .69. The assent of the subjects to the items is measured by a 5-pointed Likert scale ranging from *very inaccurate* to *very accurate*. An example item for extraversion is *I see myself as someone who is outgoing, sociable,* for agreeableness *I see myself as someone who is generally trusting,* for conscientiousness *I see myself as someone who tends to be lazy* (inverted), for neuroticism *I see myself as someone who gets nervous easily* (inverted), and for openness to experience *I see myself as someone who has an active imagination*.

Perceived Stress Questionnaire (PSQ)

To capture the feelings of anxiety based of the past 4 weeks we used the PSQ (Fliege et al. 2001). According to the manual, the 8-item-instrument shows an internal consistency (Cronbach's α) between .80 and .86. In the present study resulted .82. An example item is *I'm afraid of the future*. The participants specify their agreement to the items by a 4-pointed Likert scale ranging from *hardly ever* to *mostly*.

Emotional Intelligence

For measuring emotional intelligence, were took 12 items from the Emotional Competence Questionnaire (Rindermann 2009). The total score of these items we used to quantify emotional intelligence. An example item is *I often tell of my feelings*. The 6-pointed Likert scale ranges from *strongly disagree* to *strongly agree*. We found Cronbach's α to be .63.

Mindfulness

Mindfulness was captured by the German 12-item-version of the Kentucky Inventory of Mindfulness Skills (KIMS-D; Ströhle et al. 2010). Baer et al. (2004) found Cronbach's α to be .76. We found a value of .68. An example item is *I tend to rate my perception right or wrong*. The 7-pointed Likert scale ranges from *strongly disagree* to *strongly agree*.

3.3.3 Results

3.3.3.1 Relationships Between Art-of-Living and the Big Five

The first line of Table 3.5 presents the results, which yields: The correlation of overall art-of-living and extraversion (.42), agreeableness (.31), conscientiousness (.39), openness (.21) as well as neuroticism (−.59) show significant but not very high correlations with the art-of-living total score. It is in line with expectations that art-of-living is a kind of missing neuroticism, and it shows low to medium correlations with agreeableness, conscientiousness and extraversion. A little bit unexpected is the low correlation with openness, if one reminds that openness is part of the construct of art-of-living. A more fine grained view allows the study of the subscale relationships. We look for the highest and lowest correlation for each Big Five scale. Extraversion correlates with *openness* but not with *serenity* and *reflection*. There is a medium correlation of agreeableness with *serenity* and no correlation with *shaping of living conditions* and *reflection*. Conscientiousness shows the highest relationship with *optimization* but no correlation with *positive attitude towards life*, *serenity* and *savoring*. Neuroticism is highly negatively related to *serenity* and *self-efficacy* but only a little bit to *social contact*. That art-of-living's *openness* correlates with Big Five's openness is not surprisingly but the small amount of this relationship points to the fact that these constructs have only a small overlap but also represent different aspects. Openness has in comparison with the other Big Five factors the lowest convergence with art-of-living.

Table 3.5 Correlations of art-of-living and the BFI-K

Art-of-living	Extraversion	Agreeableness	Conscientiousness	Neuroticism	Openness
Art-of living-total	.42***	.31***	.39***	−.59***	.21***
Balance	.35***	.23***	.26***	−.44***	.16*
Coping	.25***	.18**	.35***	−.36***	.01
Serenity	.08	.37***	.00	−.69***	.14*
Savoring	.34***	.13*	.11	−.41***	.20**
Self-determined way of living	.29***	.17**	.40***	−.45***	.17**
Meaning	.34***	.30***	.29***	−.37***	.09
Social contact	.26***	.20**	.15*	−.21***	.09
Self-efficacy	.38***	.18**	.30***	−.56***	.11
Shaping of living conditions	.31***	.08	.32***	−.26***	.21***
Physical care	.19**	.13*	.36***	−.28***	.15*
Integrating different areas of living	.21***	.30***	.20**	−.51***	−.02
Openness	.46***	.25***	.28***	−.54***	.29***
Optimization	.26***	.19**	.46***	−.48***	−.06
Positive attitude towards life	.42***	.30***	.09	−.43***	.06
Reflection	.08	.07	.18**	.13*	.31***
Self-actualization	.28***	.15*	.41***	−.34***	.24***
Self-knowledge	.26***	.22***	.31***	−.30***	.23***

N = 242
*** $p < .001$; ** $p < .01$; * $p < .05$

3.3.3.2 Incremental Validity of Art-of-Living Compared to the Big Five with Respect to Well-Being

We just showed the relationships between the Big Five and art-of-living. It could be demonstrated that there are meaningful correlations. Now the question is whether all the information of art-of-living for the prediction of well-being is already contained in the Big Five so that art-of-living would not enhance the prediction.

Therefore, we perform a regression with two blocks of predictors. We first predict well-being only with the Big Five and then in addition, we include art-of-living into the prediction.

Based on the same sample as for the previous question we get the following results. The Big Five variables have a multiple correlation of $R = .61$; $R^2 = .38$; ($F = 28.5$ $df_1 = 5$, $df_2 = 236$, $p < .001$). By adding the group of art-of-living variables results $R = .84$; $R^2 = .71$ and R^2 change is .33 ($F = 14.4$; $df_1 = 17$; $df_2 = 219$, $p < .001$). That means although the Big Five show a multiple correlation of .61 with well-being, the art-of-living allows an additional significant amount (33 %) of prediction in well-being. That can be interpreted as incremental validity.

Table 3.6 Correlations between art-of-living and emotional intelligence, mindfulness and anxiety

Art-of-living	Emotional Intelligence	Mindfulness	Anxiety
Art-of-living total	.71***	.64***	−.75***
Balance	.56***	.52***	−.31***
Coping	.32***	.29***	−.37***
Serenity	.47***	.26***	−.61***
Savoring	.37***	.31***	−.64***
Integrating different areas of living	.31***	.29***	−.52***
Openness	.43***	.35***	−.32***
Optimization	.49***	.50***	−.42***
Positive attitude towards life	.55***	.52***	−.65***
Self-knowledge	.57***	.52***	−.42***
Self-determined way of living	.59***	.51***	−.56***
Social contact	.44***	.44***	−.40***
Self-efficacy	.54***	.45***	−.52***
Shaping of living conditions	.48***	.48***	−.48***

$N = 178$
*** $p < .001$

3.3.3.3 Art-of-Living and Anxiety, Emotional Intelligence and Mindfulness

Table 3.6 shows the correlative relationships between art-of-living and emotional intelligence, mindfulness and anxiety. Emotional intelligence total correlates with art of living total to .71. On the level of art-of-living subscales, the highest correlations occur for *self-determined way of living* (.59), *self-knowledge* (.57), and *balance* (.56).

Total mindfulness correlates with total art-of-living to .64. The highest correlations on subscale basis resulted for *self-knowledge, balance* and *positive attitude towards life* (all .52). In view of art-of-living, introspection (or "self-awareness") is a part of mindfulness, and introspection also is a basic tool for *self-knowledge*. So both concepts have common shares, which are reflected by the correlation.

Art-of-living total shows a correlation of −.75 with anxiety total.

3.3.4 Discussion

Art-of-living shows some systematic relationships with the Big Five. The relationship with neuroticism is highly negative and with extraversion positive and of medium size. Each art-of-living subconstruct has at least a correlation of .29 with one of the Big Five variables but besides three relationships to neuroticism there are no correlations higher than .5. In sum, there are relationships to the Big Five but they are not very high so that one can conclude, that art-of-living is more or something different than pure personality. This could be proved by the multiple regression where it could be shown that art-of-living significantly and substantially increases the predictability of well-being. In so far it seems to be justified to further investigate the construct art-of-living. The meaningful correlations with emotional intelligence and mindfulness confirm that both aspects are related to art-of-living. As expected, anxciety is negativ related with art-of-living.

3.4 Validation: Key Constructs of Positive Psychology—Ways of Leading a Good Life Relationships Between Art-of-Living and Strength and Virtues and Orientation to Happiness

Bettina Schumacher

3.4.1 *Introduction*

In Chap. 1 a conceptual overview showed that leading a good life by using art-of-living strategies should result in happiness, Sect. 3.1 provided empirical results. In the following chapter we will analyze the relationships between art-of-living and other ways of leading a good life: *strengths and virtues* and *orientation to happiness* (OTH). Whereas the constructs were described in the introduction we now turn to the kind of measurement. Therefore, strengths and virtues and orientation to happiness are explained in more detail.

3.4.1.1 Strengths and Virtues (Peterson and Seligman 2004)

Peterson and Seligman (2004) performed a comprehensive and extensive systematic review of existing catalogues of virtues in ancient and modern Eastern and Western philosophy. As main result they built broader categories of virtues: *wisdom, justice, temperance, courage, humanity* and *transcendence.* Each of these broad categories of virtues comprises a group of character strength, see Table 3.7.

Table 3.7 Virtues and their corresponding strengths according to Peterson and Seligman (2004)

Virtue	Character strengths
Wisdom & knowledge	Creativity, curiosity, open-mindedness, love of learning, perspective
Courage	Integrity, bravery, persistence, vitality
Humanity	Kindness, love, social intelligence
Justice	Fairness, leadership, citizenship
Temperance	Forgiveness and mercy, modesty and humility, prudence, self-regulation
Transcendence	Appreciation of beauty and excellence, gratitude, hope, humor, spirituality

This concept of character strengths was selected for validation since it is well established in positive psychology and in numerous studies it was shown that these strengths and virtues describe possible ways to reach well-being, cf. Chap. 1. We argue that this categorization contains some moral evaluations and that is one of the reasons why we prefer the concept art-of-living. A further difference to the concept of art-of-living is that virtues and strength are at least partially determined by inborn traits whereas art-of-living conceptualized as attitudes and strategies are more the result of experience and learning. But it is very interesting to study both their communalities and differences in detail.

3.4.1.2 Orientation to Happiness

The orientation to happiness comprises three fundamentally different attitudes towards life (Seligman 2002), that is the "life motto" or philosophy of life. Each of these attitudes is unique in the way it enables people to achieve a fulfilling life with a qualitatively different potential. The first aspect, the *life of pleasure,* follows the hedonistic principle of maximizing enjoyment and minimizing suffering. The *life of engagement* however is implemented by engaging in fulfilling activities in which one can become completely absorbed. This OTH component is related to the concept of *flow* by Csikszentmihalyi (1990). Lastly, the *life of meaning,* based on an eudaimonic approach, is characterized by finding meaning in one's life by dedicating the latter to a higher purpose. Comparing orientation to happiness and art-of-living they are both resource-oriented, relevant for the everyday life and focus on the enhancement of individual well-being. While the philosophy of life (OTH) defines a more general attitude towards life, the art-of-living is far more differentiated and focuses on applicable strategies related to the subcomponents.

3.4.2 Method

3.4.2.1 Sample

The sample collected by Schumacher (2015) comprised 636 participants and is described more in detail in Sect. 3.1.2.1.

3.4.2.2 Instruments

Art-of-Living

The revised version of the art-of-living-questionnaire (see Sect. 2.4) was applied.

Short Version of the Values in Action Inventory of Strengths (VIA-24)

In order to measure character strengths in the present study was used a 24 item short version (VIA-24) by Furnham and Lester (2012), which contains one item per character strengths. The internal consistency (Cronbach's α) of the total scale[1] calculated in the study of Schumacher (2015) is .80. For answering items the subjects should assess the extent of the own character strengths compared to the general public. Therefore it was a 5-pointed Likert scale available which ranged from *well below the average* to *well above average*. An example item for wisdom ($\alpha = .66$) is *Curiosity: interest in, intrigued by many things*, one for courage ($\alpha = .55$) is *Bravery: courage, valor, fearlessness*, one for love ($\alpha = .52$) is *Kindness: generosity, empathic, helpful*, one for justice ($\alpha = .48$) is *Citizenship: team worker, loyalty, duty to others*, one for temperance ($\alpha = .55$) is *Self-control: able to regulate emotions, nonimpulsive*, and one for transcendence ($\alpha = .76$) is *Appreciative of beauty: seeking excellence, experience of awe/wonder.*

Orientation to Happiness (OTH)

The three factor construct for measuring the orientation to happiness was designed by Peterson et al. (2005) and registers each of the three philosophies of life with six items respectively. The internal consistency (Cronbach's α) of the total scale calculated in the study of Schumacher (2015) was .74. For the subscales arose .74 for life of pleasure, .70 for life of engagement and .71 for life of meaning. Peterson et al. (2005) found internal consistencies of .82 for life of pleasure, .72 for life of engagement and .82 for life of meaning. The internal consistencies of the subscales thus could be replicated in the study of Schumacher (2015) roughly. The consent of the subjects to the items was recorded with a 5-pointed Likert scale, ranging from *very much unlike me* until *very much like me.* A sample item for life of engagement is *I am always very absorbed in what I do*; for life of pleasure *Life is too short to postpone the pleasures it can provide*; for life of meaning *I have a responsibility to make the world a better place.*

3.4.3 Results

3.4.3.1 Art-of-Living and Strengths and Virtues

Table 3.8 contains the correlations between art-of-living and the VIA strengths and virtues. Note that due to the low Cronbach's α of some VIA-components, we will

[1]Furnham and Lester (2012) do not report Cronbach's α for the total scale.

Table 3.8 Correlations of art-of-living and strengths and virtues as well as orientation to happiness

Art-of-living questionnaire (ALQ)	Strengths and virtues (VIA-24)							Orientation to Happiness (OTH)			
	Justice[a]	Love[a]	Temperance[a]	Courage[a]	Transcendence	Wisdom	VIA-24 total	Pleasure	Engagement	Meaning	OTH total
Art-of-living total	.34***	.30***	.12**	.39***	.55***	.44***	.59***	.39***	.50***	.37***	.58***
Balance	.29***	.33***	.03	.23***	.44***	.32***	.45***	.32***	.38***	.23***	.43***
Coping	.27***	.16***	.18***	.30***	.37***	.33***	.44***	.20***	.45***	.24***	.40***
Serenity	.11**	.05	.30***	.20***	.25***	.21***	.31***	.04	.24***	.09*	.16***
Savoring	.13**	.17***	.01	.08*	.43***	.22***	.54***	.44***	.29***	.17***	.41***
Self-determined way of living	.22***	.14***	.03	.39***	.31***	.34***	.30***	.24***	.36***	.21***	.37***
Meaning	.26***	.30***	.03	.33***	.46***	.26***	.45***	.35***	.43***	.41***	.56***
Social contact	.28***	.41***	.05	.18***	.34***	.15***	.35***	.28***	.24***	.18***	.32***
Self-efficacy	.29***	.18***	.11**	.43***	.45***	.44***	.53***	.26***	.44***	.26***	.44***
Shaping of living conditions	.17***	.14***	.00	.21***	.29***	.24***	.30***	.36***	.30***	.18***	.52***
Physical care	.15***	.11**	.08*	.24***	.25***	.22***	.29***	.21***	.21***	.25***	.32***
Integrating different areas of living	.17***	.10*	.11**	.09*	.26***	.15***	.24***	.26***	.22***	.12**	.27***
Openness	.25***	.16***	.03	.32***	.44***	.51***	.45***	.21***	.35***	.32***	.41***
Optimization	.29***	.21***	.14***	.43***	.32***	.35***	.48***	.19***	.40***	.17***	.34***
Positive attitude towards life	.24***	.29***	.07	.22***	.58***	.24***	.47***	.40***	.39***	.34***	.52***
Reflection	.14***	.04***	.14***	.03	.07	.24***	.18***	.08	.11***	.25***	.22***
Self-actualization	.27***	.22***	.02	.35***	.41***	.42***	.47***	.33***	.42**	.36***	.52***
Self-knowledge	.35***	.30***	.11**	.39***	.42***	.46***	.54***	.28***	.40***	.30***	.45***

$N = 636$
* $p < .05$; ** $p < .01$; *** $p < .001$
[a]Scale shows low reliability ($\alpha < .56$)

concentrate on the overall VIA-scale and the most reliable components: wisdom and transcendence.

Following the results of Table 3.8 we see that the highest relationships between overall art-of-living and strength and virtues are found for transcendence (.55) and wisdom (.44). Looking at details of the subscales transcendence shows higher correlations to *positive attitude towards life* and to *meaning* whereas wisdom is correlated to *openness*, *self-efficacy* and *self-actualization* and *self-knowledge*. Although we will try not to overinterpret correlations of justice, humanity, temperance and courage in detail because their low consistency it seems interesting that justice has a comparable high relationship to *balance*, humanity to *social contact*, temperance to *serenity* and courage to *self-efficacy*. In sum these relationships seem to make sense. The correlation between the overall art-of-living and overall strengths and virtues turns out to be .59, which again shows a large overlap but also that these constructs differ substantially.

Correlations of Art-of-Living with Orientation to Happiness (OTH)

The relationships between art-of-living and OTH are listed also in Table 3.8.

Most of these correlations were significant and of medium size. Life of pleasure (OTH) shows its highest relationship with *savoring* (art-of-living), life of engagement (OTH) shows the highest correlations with *coping* and *self-efficacy* (art-of-living), whereas life of meaning (OTH) correlates with *meaning* (art-of-living), which can be seen as validation although the concepts with similar labels do not seem to be totally equivalent. This might be due to the fact that OTH necessarily includes broader and more general constructs than art-of-living. Interestingly, although there is no specific construct belonging to art-of-living which represents engagement, the relationship for engagement and overall art-of-living is .50 and it is higher than the correlations of life of pleasure (OTH) with overall art-of-living and life of meaning (OTH) with overall art-of-living. Total art-of-living correlates with total OTH significant to .58.

3.4.4 Discussion

The sample for validation is quite large, the subscales of art-of-living and OTH can be reliable measured as well as some of the virtues and strength, namely transcendence, wisdom and the overall virtues.

In sum, the conclusion regarding the relationships of art-of-living with OTH is similar than with respect to virtues and strength and art-of-living: there are meaningful overlaps and substantial differences which support the usefulness of the development of art-of-living.

3.5 Validation: Related Constructs—Resilience, Coherence, Self-Regulation and Wisdom and Their Relationships to the Art-of-Living

Anne Traulsen, Anna Schmidt, Bernhard Schmitz

3.5.1 Introduction

To further validate the new instrument, we used important related constructs: resilience, sense of coherence, self-regulation, and wisdom. The concepts of resilience, sense of coherence and self-regulation focus on resources and protective factors as well as the identification of factors that contribute to the development and maintenance of mental and physical health (Fröhlich-Gildhoff and Rönnau-Böse 2009). Wisdom is connected with adequate judging and action and is seen as a way to provide the individual and society with a good life even in the case of uncertainties (Kekes 1988; Maxwell 2004; Thiele 2006). Resilience, sense of coherence, self-regulation, wisdom, and the art-of-living as we describe it, are thus concepts that broadly and positively influence life and its individual arrangement. We consider these concepts to be appropriate for further validation, and thus, we test whether there are positive correlations between them and art-of-living.

3.5.1.1 Resilience

Generally, resilience can be defined as a person's mental capability of resistance (Knoll et al. 2011). It dates back to a long-term study conducted by Emmy Werner (1993) analyzing a sample of Hawaiian children, many of which matured excellently despite being subjected to various risk factors endangering a healthy development. Resilience can also be regarded as the opposite of vulnerability (Schumacher et al. 2004). The following study measured resilience as a trait.

3.5.1.2 Sense of Coherence

The SOC can be defined as "the extent to which one has a pervasive, enduring though dynamic, feeling of confidence that one's environment is predictable and that things will work out as well as can reasonably be expected" (Antonovsky 1987). According to Antonovsky (1987) this feeling of confidence comprises three aspects:

1. Stimuli resulting from both the inner and outer environment over the lifespan show a comprehensible structure, are predictable and explainable.
2. The resources required in order to fulfill these stimuli's demands are available.
3. These demands represent challenges worth effort and endeavor.

The higher a person's sense of coherence is, the easier it is to remain healthy. An individual with a strong sense of coherence usually finds it easier to adapt dynamically to requirements, whereas a counterpart with low coherence might strive to fulfill the requirements following a strict routine, not accessing or perceiving further resources (Bengel et al. 2001).

3.5.1.3 Self-Regulation

It is not obvious that self-regulation is related to art-of-living. Therefore, we want to elaborate on the relationship. In short, self-regulation is defined as the pursuing of self-set goals (cf. Zimmerman et al. 2000; Schmitz and Wiese 2006) whereas art-of-living is the living of a self-determined life. Art-of-living is a much broader concept than self-regulation. Art-of-living for example contains savoring and positive attitude towards life which are not components of self-regulation. Common parts are optimization and reflection. These communalities make it interesting to study the empirical overlapping. We expect a medium correlation between both constructs.

3.5.1.4 Wisdom

Wisdom is probably present in most people's mundane vocabulary. But what is wise exactly? Originating in a divine context this attribute was transferred to humanity via ancient Greek philosophers like Socrates, Plato and Aristotle. Wisdom was understood as knowledge and judgement (Baltes and Kunzmann 2003). Although many philosophers analyzed the nature, the development and the function of wisdom since then, most approaches were theoretical or speculative (Baltes et al. 1995). It was not until the 1980s that psychologists began to analyze this topic. Preceding studies in the field of lifespan psychology inspired this research (Baltes and Kunzmann 2003). In this context, wisdom was regarded as an "ideal final stage of human development" and therefore analyzed mostly in samples of the elderly with regard to interactions between wisdom, experience and understandings acquired over the lifespan.

> We do not receive wisdom, we must discover it for ourselves, after a journey through the wilderness which no one else can make for us, which no one can spare us, for our wisdom is the point of view from which we come at last to regard the world. (Marcel Proust 1990).

Empirical Approach to Measure Individual Wisdom

Over the last decades two approaches proved particularly successful in wisdom research. There is also an important approach from Sternberg (1998). The models described in the following paragraphs are the Berlin Wisdom Paradigm created by Paul Baltes and his research team and the Three-Dimensional Wisdom Scale by Monika Ardelt (2003).

The Berlin Wisdom Paradigm

Paul Baltes and his colleagues assumed that wisdom represents the ability to come to satisfactory decisions on important problems in life and to be able to give advice (Staudinger et al. 1992). This construct's most important central aspect is *knowledge.* The model comprises five criteria of wisdom, two basic- and three meta-criteria. The former are:

(a) An extensive declarative knowledge on various circumstances and the course of life (e.g. the nature of humans, emotions, motives) and
(b) A rich procedural knowledge about coping-strategies for various problems in life (e.g. strategies to come to a satisfactory decision) (Baltes and Smith 2008).

The first meta-criterion is the so called lifespan-contextualism. It describes knowing that a persons' attitudes and behavior should be contemplated and judged not isolated but in the context of age, cultural background and individual history (Baltes and Smith 2008; Staudinger et al. 1992). The second meta-criterion—the value-relativism—is closely related to the lifespan-contextualism. It describes being aware that individual values, goals and priorities strongly depend on personality traits and the cultural background. Finally, the last meta-criterion comprised by the Berlin Wisdom-Paradigm focuses on knowledge about strategies for coping with life's uncertainty and unpredictability (Baltes and Smith 2008). Positively managing these aspects can—according to the model—be described as making assumptions about future events and developments, making the best possible decisions and trusting one's judgement while not ignoring the fact that the decisions suitability and applicability might have to be reappraised later. The intention behind the corresponding instrument is to confront subjects with difficult hypothetical situations illustrating fictional characters' problems or dilemmas, about which participants are instructed to think and comment verbally (Baltes et al. 1995; Staudinger et al. 1992). For instance, one situation described a 15 year old girl intending to marry immediately. The answer was rated as wise if it achieved high scores in all five categories (Baltes et al. 1995; Staudinger et al. 1992).

The Three-Dimensional Wisdom Scale (3D-WS)

Monika Ardelt (2003) regards wisdom as a personal characteristic. Consequently, she does not utilize fictitious scenarios but rather measures a person's behaviors and attitudes with her questionnaire. Wisdom, according to her, is not a parameter based solely on knowledge as is assumed by Baltes and his colleagues (Baltes et al. 1995; Baltes and Smith 1990; Baltes and Staudinger 1993), but rather a latent variable comprising both a cognitive as well as a reflexive component. Items associated with the cognitive component of wisdom are designed to measure the subjects' ability and willingness to comprehend a situation or phenomenon completely (Ardelt 2003). An inverted sample item describes striving for profound understanding as follows: "Simply knowing the answer rather than understanding the reasons for the answer to a problem is fine with me." On the other hand, the reflexive dimension focuses on the ability to and intention of analyzing the environment from various perspectives and thereby generating distance from the personal point of view, also included are items concerning attribution, i.e. measuring the degree to which participants regard either their environment or themselves as responsible for their situation. Sample item: *I always try to look at all sides of a problem.*

Lastly, the affective dimension completes Ardelt's model of wisdom. It is associated with empathy and compassion for others. More specifically it measures the presence of positive, negative or neutral emotions and behaviors. Inverted example: *It's not really my problem if others are in trouble and need help.*

3.5.2 Method

3.5.2.1 Sample

For analyzing the relationship to art-of-living the following samples (see Chap. 2) are used:

For resilience and sense of coherence: Partial sample A included 158 participants, the majority was female (66.50 %) with a mean age of 39.50 years (SD = 12.55). Most participants were in a relationship (34.80 %) or married (33.50 %). 26.6 % were single, 3.8 % divorced, and 2 widowed. To have one child at least 38.60 % of the participants stated.

For self-regulation: Partial sample B was collected during a lesson. The students were asked to work on the questionnaires regarding art-of-living and self-regulation. A group of 71 students took part which has similar characteristics as other German students of humanities.

For wisdom: Partial sample C (N = 204) again was predominantly female (66.20 %) with a mean age of 26.30 years (SD = 9.43 %). Again, most participants stated to be in a relationship (48.00 %). A stuck of 11.30 % was married, 39.70 % were single. 1.00 % was divorced. 11.30 % stated to have one child at least.

Samples A and C are subsamples of the entire sample (N = 1105) which is described more in detail in Chap. 2.

3.5.2.2 Instruments

In addition to the original form art-of-living-questionnaire (see Chap. 2) and the satisfaction with life scale (see Chap. 2) the following questionnaires were used:

Resilience Scale (RS-11)

In order to measure resilience, an abridged edition of the German version of Wagnild and Young's (1993) resilience scale with eleven items (RS-11) was used. Answers were reported using a 7-pointed Likert scale ranging from *complete agreement* to *complete disagreement* (Schumacher et al. 2004). A sample item is *I usually cope with this one way or another.* According to Schumacher et al. (2004), Cronbach's α is .91.

Sense of Coherence Scale (SOC-13)

SOC-13 (Schumacher et al. 2000) comprises 13 Items, e.g.: *Do you feel like you don't actually care for what happens in your environment?* Subjects responded using a 7-pointed Likert scale from *rarely or never* to *very frequently.* According to Schumacher et al. (2000), Cronbach's α is .85.

Self-Regulation Questionnaire

We applied eigth scales of the self-regulation questionnaire from Bellhäuser, Roth and Schmitz (2015), namely: *reflection* (α = .75, we found .68), *time-management* (α = .64, we found .66), *metacognition* (α = .61, we found .58), *procrastination* (α = .70, we found .79), *motivation* (α = .66, we found .64), *goal-setting* (α = .67, we found .72), *self-instruction* (α = .73, we found .77) and *social learning* (α = .61, we found .72). The internal consistency of the total scale is α = .87, we found .91. An example item for the scale *reflection* is *At the end of the day I ask myself if I'm satisfied with my performance.* Altogether, it consists of 62 items. To the subjects there is a 6-pointed Likert scale available ranging from *correct* to *not correct.*

The 3D-WS for Measuring Wisdom

Ardelt's (2006) German version contains 39 items associated with a cognitive (14), a reflexive (13) and an affective (12) dimension measuring responses using a 5-pointed Likert scale ranging from *definitely true of myself* to *not true to myself* for the first part of the questionnaire and ranging from *strongly agree* to *strongly disagree* for the second part of the questionnaire. The first part has a reference to the own personality, the second part describes generally statements. A sample item is *I always try to look at all sides of a problem.* Cronbach's α values for the cognitive, reflective, and affective dimensions were .78, .75, and .74 (for the follow-up after 10 months .85, .71, and .72).

3.5.3 Results

Correlative analyses were conducted in order to examine the relationships between the art-of-living and the related constructs resilience, coherence, self-regulation, and wisdom, s. Table 3.9. For resilience a correlation of .68 with total art-of-living reveals.

Sense of coherence shows a similar correlation of .69.

The total scores of self-regulation and art-of-living correlates to .61.

Table 3.9 Correlations of art-of-living with resilience, sense of coherence, self-regulation and wisdom

	Resilience[a]	Coherence[a]	Self-regulation[b]	Wisdom[c]
Art-of-living total	.68***	.69***	.61***	.58***
Balance	.52***	.37***	.39***	.34***
Coping	.44***	.43***	.60***	.39***
Serenity	.22**	.53***	.14	.50***
Savoring	.20*	.23**	.27*	.17*
Self-determined way of living	.54***	.59***	.58***	.50***
Social contact	.45***	.42***	.35**	.46***
Self-efficacy	.53***	.40***	.40***	.37***
Shaping of living conditions	.37***	.34***	.40***	.32***
Physical care	.33***	.27***	.41***	.25***
Integrating different areas of living	.24**	.37***	.43***	.35***
Openness	.52***	.45***	.35**	.41***
Optimization	.47***	.43***	.62***	.41***
Positive attitude towards life	.48***	.51***	.28**	.45***
Self-knowledge	.57***	.47***	.55***	.33***

* $p < .05$; ** $p < .01$; *** $p < .001$

[a]$n = 158$ (Schmitz and Schmidt 2014)

[b]$n = 71$ (Student Sample 2015)

[c]$n = 204$ (Schmitz and Schmidt 2014)

Likewise, wisdom and the art-of-living also correlate moderately to highly. The overall correlation amounted to .58, while the art-of-living scales *self-determined way of living* and *serenity* show the highest relationship (both .50). However, it is assumed that the high correlation between wisdom and the art-of-living can be attributed to the reflexive dimension in particular. Therefore we computed the relationship of art-of-living with the overall scale of wisdom and its subscales: cognitive wisdom, reflexive wisdom and affective wisdom. The analyses revealed the following significant correlations: .57 for the overall scale, .36 for the cognitive .67, for the reflexive, and .33 for the affective component of wisdom, respectively. Looking at the subscales of art-of-living (cf. Table 3.9) the highest relationship of resilience is with *self-knowledge* and *self-determined way of living* whereas *savoring* has the lowest relationship with resilience, coherence and wisdom. Interestingly coherence has high correlations in addition to *self-determined way of living,* to *positive attitude towards life* and *serenity.* Wisdom is highly related to *self-determined way of living* and *serenity.* The correlations to the overall score of art-of-living are higher than for each subscale which can be interpreted that the combination of art-of-living sub-constructs is of special importance.

In sum, the expected correlations between the art-of-living and its related constructs wisdom, resilience, self-regulation and coherence were confirmed.

3.6 Art-of-Living: Measuring the Construct Using the Situational Judgement Test

Carolin Rupp, Magdalena Krankenhagen, Janina Linten

3.6.1 Introduction

When intending to measure art-of-living, a questionnaire seems to be the most obvious way. The problems when using questionnaires are well known. It is difficult to avoid effects of social desirability (Kelava and Moosbrugger 2012) and also to take into account effects of situational dependency. Questionnaires are supposed to measure more intentions for behavior than real behavior. All these problems let researchers to the development of Situational Judgement Tests, which are intended to avoid problems of social desirability, situation effects and unprecise measurement of behavior (Bledow and Frese 2009).

3.6.1.1 What Is a Situational Judgement Test (SJT)?

The SJT is a questionnaire confronting participants with descriptions of situations, asking them to state how they would behave in the respective scenario (Bledow and Frese 2009). For each situation various response options are provided. The participants are asked to imagine the described scene before deciding for the behavior which they would probably show within this situation. Because in this way of measurement different kinds of situations can be included and the response options describe behavior, the problems of situation effects and inappropriate behavior measurement are reduced. Also because the subjects cannot detect easily which answer option seems to be related to the construct under investigation the possibility of *socially desirable* answers is reduced. Therefore in a series of studies we try to develop an SJT for art-of-living. The presented scenarios should describe every-day situations in which art-of-living behavior could be observable. The test at hand is based on Bledow's and Freses's statements (2009) on designing an SJT and is a revised version of the art-of-living-SJT by Rupp (2014) which is based on Bending's test (2013).

3.6.2 *Method*

3.6.2.1 Sample

Two samples were used:

The sample recorded by Rupp (2014) includes 103 subjects, thereof 55.4 % females. 89.3 % stated to be unmarried, 9.7 % to be married and 1 % to be divorced.

The sample recorded by Krankenhagen (2015) includes 153 subjects with a stuck of 53.6 % females. The mean age was 27.88 years (*SD* = 7.49). The youngest was 17, the oldest 66 years old. 42.5 % reported to be single, 12.4 % married, 2 % divorced and 43.1 % to have a relationship.

3.6.2.2 Instruments

Well-Being

We use the SWLS, the satisfaction with life scale (Diener et al. 1985) cf. Chap. 2.

Happiness

In addition we apply the SHS, the subjective happiness scale (Lyubomirsky 2008), cf. above.

Art-of-Living-Questionnaire

For the revised art-of-living-questionnaire, see Chap. 2.

Art-of-Living SJT

This instrument is newly developed in this study.

The basis for the *Situational Judgement Test* was provided by Schmitz' and Schmidt's (2014) questionnaire. We tried to measure each subconstruct with a few items.

The excerpts from the Situational Judgement Test provided in the upcoming paragraphs are designed to illustrate the questionnaire's structure. We decided to build four response options. One option which is not related to the construct and therefore is assigned a value of 0. Two answer options which seem to be a little bit fitting to the construct, which were assigned a value of 1, and finally an option which fits very good to the construct which is assigned a value of 3.

Example 1 regarding the scale o*penness.*

A friend took you to a group for the first time, e.g. yoga class, soccer team, choir etc.

- *You would like to get to know the still unacquainted people better, have a pleasant conversation and appreciate the new contacts.* 3
- *If it arises out of the situation you will start talking to the others.* 1
- *As your friend is the only person you know, you mostly talk to him at first.* 1
- *You have come here to participate in the group. Someday an opportunity presents itself you will get to know the others better.* 0

Example 2 regarding the scale *coping.*

During a meeting you received critical feedback…

- *You are uncomfortable with the fact of having made a mistake. You hope to avoid it in the future.* 1
- *You find it unpleasant, however you know how to behave more adequate next time.* 3
- *Everyone makes mistakes. You decide to make an effort to make less mistakes next time.* 1
- *You cannot understand how this could have happened and feel angry towards yourself.* 0

In summary, the SJT contains 61 items representing all subconstructs of art-of-living.

The internal consistency of the total scores of the SJT is $\alpha = .73$, which is not very high, but in line with SJT for other constructs, cf. Bledow and Frese (2009).

3.6.3 Results

A correlation between art-of-living and art-of-living SJT was found (.56). Both measures, the art-of-living SJT and the art-of-living-questionnaire show a significant positive correlation with the well-being/happiness measures: art-of-living SJT with SWLS, SHS .15, .27, whereas art-of-living questionnaire correlates with SWLS, SHS to .53, .51.

3.6.4 Discussion

In this study it was tried to develop a SJT for art-of-living. The results show that important first steps were made, but that the SJT art-of-living is yet in a preparation stage. But with respect to the validation of the art-of-living questionnaire the SJT is an additional instrument to capture art-of-living. In sum art-of-living can be measured in different ways, with a suitable consistency at least at the overall scale level.

3.7 Validity of Self- and Peer-Assessment for the Art-of-Living

Nafiseh Küffner

3.7.1 Introduction

In personality research, instruments of self-assessment are often used to measure a number of personality traits. Next to the economic application, an important advantage of such an operationalization is the possibility to measure experiences which cannot be accessed any other way. Since these reports are based on subjective answers, they can be affected by biases which are, among others, caused by self-deception or deliberate self-portrayal (Weber and Rammsayer 2012). Another fundamental problem of this kind of operationalization is whether these assessments are even valid and accurately reflect the person's traits (Spinath 2000). However, methods which rely on more objective data can also be considered for the validation of psychological constructs. For this, the construct validity of self-assessment is validated with peer-assessment (Paunonen and Oneill 2010). Recently, Ruch et al. (2010) have validated the German adaption of the questionnaire for the assessment of character strengths and virtues by Peterson et al. (2005) with peer-assessments and have found a medium correlation of .40. Other studies about well-being showed medium correlations between .28 and .36 (Watson and Clark 1991). Very high correlations are usually not expected, since the person assessing him- or herself has access to information from earlier experiences as well as to thoughts, feelings and motives the peer-evaluator does not have. Therefore it is assumed that the degree of correspondence increases with the time the peer-evaluator has known the person and the amount of information he or she has about the evaluated person (Amelang et al. 2006). In this light, results from studies in which unfamiliar people are asked to judge a person about whom they have only minimal information can be used as a comparison. They show significant correlations (from .05 to .42; Paunonen and Oneill 2010), but the correlations between self- and peer-assessment by a partner or a friend are higher. (Borkenau et al. 2011, Costa and McCrae 1992a, b). Funder and Colvin (1988) argues that the constant observation of a person's behavior both by the person as well as by an acquaintance leads to respective self- and peer-concepts. Therefore the peer-concepts are the more differentiated the longer the two have known each other.

The accuracy of the correspondence depends, among others, on the possibility to observe the evaluated traits (Amelang et al. 2006). A study about the assessment of the observability of traits shows that traits which can be observed very well have a positive correlation with extraversion and a negative with neuroticism (Funder and Dobroth 1987). The authors assume that traits from the field of extraversion can be observed directly in the social behavior of a person and are therefore easier to judge, whereas this is not true for traits regarding emotional stability (Funder and Dobroth 1987). Peer-evaluators judge a person less biased and more objectively with regard to social desired traits (Paunonen and Oneill 2010). According to Ruch et al. (2010) it is assumed that self-evaluators tend to overestimation when judging their own personality aspects and that therefore there would be significant differences in the means of scales of self- and peer-assessment. According to Schahn and Amelang (1992) significant differences in these means are especially found with items influenced by social desirability and not with dimensions which are neutral regarding social desirability.

We assume that the relationship between self- and peer-assessment of art-of-living will be significant but not very high. It is expected that the mean of the peer-assessment is significantly lower than the mean of the self-assessment.

3.7.2 *Method*

3.7.2.1 Sample

The sample consists of each 100 self- and peer-evaluators. 55 self-evaluators were male and 45 female. The mean age was 32.33 years (SD = 14.64). 40 participants reported the General Certificate of Secondary Education as highest degree, 27 reported to have a university degree. 45 were single, 24 in a relationship, 25 married and 5 divorced.

The peer-evaluator's sample was acquired by the participants themselves. 56 of them were male and 44 female. Their mean age was 30.24 years (SD = 13.48). In average the number of years the self- and the peer-evaluators know each other amounted to 8.09. 59 of the peer-evaluators reported a friendship as relationship form, 16 were married, 8 were in a relationship. The remaining relationship forms were of familial nature.

3.7.2.2 Instruments

Every self-evaluator was given the revised questionnaire about art-of-living (see Chap. 2) for the self- as well as the peer-assessment. The questionnaire for peer-assessment consists of the exact same scales and the items as the instrument for self-assessment. For this, the questions were formulated in the third person. The items are answered on a 6-pointed Likert scale (*not true at all* to *absolutely true*) just like in the original questionnaire. A self-rating item from the scale social contact is: *I am engaged in social contacts and friendships.* The peer-rating form is *He/she is engaged in his/hers social contacts and friendships.*

3.7.3 Results

3.7.3.1 Relationship Between Self- and Peer-Assessment of Art-of-Living

An overview of the relationships between self- and peer-assessment of art-of-living is shown in Table 3.10. The resulting correlation between the over-all self- and peer-assessment is .38 and significant, and can be regarded as medium.

3.7.3.2 Comparison of Self- and Peer-Assessment Regarding Their Level

At first a repeated-measures MANOVA with the factors the art-of-living scales and self- versus peer-assessment was calculated for this purpose. The result was a significant interaction of $\Lambda = .634$, $F(17.83) = 2.823$, $p = .001$, $\eta^2 = .37$.

Next it was examined with a dependent t-test for the total score of art-of-living whether self-evaluators ($M = 4.52$, $SD = .43$, $N = 100$) and peer-evaluators ($M = 4.39$, $SD = .54$, $N = 100$) differ significantly regarding their means. The t test resulted in a significant difference between the means of the two groups with $t(99) = 22.82, p = .025, d = .26$, which is considered a small effect size after Cohen (1988). That means overall self-evaluators give higher evaluations then their peers. This result can be confirmed by looking at the comparisons of the subscales for peer- and self-assessment which show differences for the most scales.

Table 3.10 Descriptive statistics, reliability and correlation between self- and peer-assessment of art-of-living

Art-of-living	Self-assessment			Peer-assessment			Self/peer
	M	*SD*	*A*	*M*	*SD*	α	*r*
Art-of-living total	4.52	.43	.97	4.39	.54	96	.38***
Balance	4.56	.58	.43	4.39	.65	59	.13
Coping	4.07	.75	.65	3.77	.80	70	.30**
Serenity	3.41	.94	.70	3.5	.99	76	.20
Savoring	4.35	.68	.64	4.28	.73	67	.44***
Self-determined way of living	4.55	.68	.68	4.43	.74	73	.10
Meaning	4.92	.63	.85	4.76	.70	87	.35***
Social contact	4.81	.63	.72	4.86	.95	55	.25**
Self-efficacy	4.46	.63	.80	4.4	.71	86	.19
Shaping of living conditions	4.77	.73	.79	4.53	.85	84	.35***
Physical care	4.33	.85	.83	4.3	1.13	88	.44***
Integrating different areas of living	3.98	.75	.50	4.1	.80	61	.28**
Openess	4.34	.61	.53	4.17	.77	73	.32**
Optimization	4.36	.61	.68	4.26	.64	73	.32**
Positive attitude towards life	4.71	.62	.74	4.61	.75	85	.43***
Reflection	4.59	.69	.77	4.24	.97	34	.28**
Self-actualization	4.91	.58	.75	4.69	.71	85	.40***
Self-knowledge	4.80	.61	.82	4.62	.70	89	.25**

N = 100 self-evaluators. N = 100 peer-evaluators
* $p < .05$; ** $p < .01$

3.7.4 Discussion

In summary, the medium-sized relationship of the art-of-living instruments (self- and peer-assessment) can be confirmed. With that the assumption of convergent validity is met for the most part, since different kinds of operationalization of the same construct lead to comparable results (Borkenau et al. 2011)

The difficulty regarding a more complicated observation of several traits (Buschor et al. 2013) by peer-evaluators could also have played a role in this study, as certain aspects of art-of-living are not necessarily apparent to an outsider.

Looking at the correlations in Table 3.10, there are subconstructs for which the self-and peer-assessments co-vary and some for which they do not. The highest correlations were found for *savoring*, *physical care* and *positive attitude towards life*, whereas those for *balance*, *serenity*, *self-efficacy* and *self-determined way of living* were not significant. This is in line with the assumption about the observability of the constructs, e.g. savoring and physical care can be observed quite easily whereas complex constructs such as balance and self-efficacy are more difficult to detect from the outside. But what is important for our purpose is that these assessments correspond and that not all answers can be attributed to social desirability or to random answers.

3.8 Art-of-Living in Working Life

Victoria Misch, Bettina Schumacher

3.8.1 Introduction

3.8.1.1 Working from the Perspective of Art-of-Living

Organizational Psychology also benefits from Positive Psychology research. Companies have started to integrate Positive Psychology elements in everyday work. At least since Herzberg (e.g. see Herzberg et al. 1959), the focus of personal development is moving away from pure hygiene factors like income, leadership and job security toward motivational factors like personal growth, responsibility and achievement. The research by Wrzesniewski et al. (1997) shows, that indeed each work has the potential to contribute to one's well-being, and that the extent of fulfilment experienced at work depends to a non-negligible part on the inner attitude. Thus, workers who consider their task not as pure duty, money source or one way to receive prestige, but as higher mission are more satisfied and show better performance. A suitable means to influence the worker's attitude is *job crafting* (Berg et al. 2013; Hackman and Oldham 1980; Grant 2007). Job crafting means the active shaping of the job tasks through the worker itself in that way, that he or she perceive the task as more interesting, meaningful and fulfilling, which leads to enhanced motivation, happiness and improved performance.

As already explained, the active shaping of living conditions is one component of the art-of-living concept. From the perspective of art-of-living, work shouldn't be considered in isolation but as an act of designing life, realization of potentials, and as pursuit of excellence. Thus, working life represents specific space for self-fulfillment. Accordingly, we consider self-fulfillment in working life as a special domain of art-of-living. The present study aims to capture the relationships between art-of-living and self-fulfillment in working life as well as components of subjective occupational success.

3.8.1.2 Self-Fulfillment in Working Life

According to Nafziger (2001, S. 84) we define self-fulfillment in working life as development of skills and traits in specific business contexts. For capturing self-fulfillment in working life we rely on the compendium *Self-fulfilment in working life* (Müller 2003), which combines recent findings from the Motivational, Cognitive, Emotional, and Organizational Psychology. The affective, cognitive, motivational, and behavioral basics of self-fulfillment in working life are self-belief, self-worth management, self-motivation, and self-promotion. In the following, we encircle this terms more exactly.

Bierhoff and Herner (2003, p. 85) define self-belief as a cognitive skill which supports goal achievement. They use the term self-efficacy synonymously. Self-efficacy describes subjective certainty, to be able to manage new or demanding tasks due to own competences. Self-efficacy in general conception was captured by Bandura (1977) for the first time. For our request, a transference of the general self-efficacy into the working life is required. This was contributed by Stief (2001) which understands vocational self-efficacy as conviction to own job specific key skills.

According to Kanning (2003), the process of self-worth management is a general interest of human beings in development and maintaining of positive self-worth which contributes, if successful, to physical and psychological health. Every person has different kinds of self-worth, for example collective and individual, private and public, and organizational self-worth. The organizational self-worth requires room to unfold ideas, wishes and potentials.

The term self-motivation stands for processes, in which a person uses consciously certain ways and means to realize own intentions. Self-motivation can also be described as active shaping of environment and self in sense of goal achievement.

Self-promotion means the ability to create a positive impression of oneself (Brand 2003). Due to the resulting reputation through others, self-promotion serves the personal development and should be practiced in certain vocational contexts. As a concrete self-promotion strategy, Bozeman and Kacmar (1997) name inter alia presenting oneself optional as exemplary or unpretentious consciously.

3.8.1.3 Components of Subjective Occupational Success

Subjective occupational success is the sum of perceived outcomes, which a person has achieved in its working life time (Judge et al. 1999). Abele et al. (2011) make a subdivision in self-referred and other-referred occupational success. Based on the conception of Dette et al. (2004) we used following criteria for capturing subjective occupational success: career satisfaction, success compared with colleagues, vocational identity, and global job satisfaction.

Lounsbury et al. (2003) define Career satisfaction "as the individual's feelings of satisfaction with his or her career as a whole" (p. 287). Comparing one's own success with colleagues, the colleagues serve as reference point.

Mieg and Woschnack (2002) emphasize, that the interaction process between work experience and identity can be regarded as development of personality. Moser and Schuler (1993) describe the vocational identity as psychological identification of a human with its profession.

There isn't any uniformly definition of global job satisfaction available (Mertel 2006). Determinants of the global job satisfaction are personality specific characteristics, characteristics of the working situation and the interaction of both.

It should be noted, that there isn't a comprehensive measurement instrument for self-fulfillment in working life available, hence we developed a new instrument based on the findings of Müller (2003) which combines single aspects of self-fulfillment in working life. These single aspects are explained below.

3.8.2 *Method*

3.8.2.1 Sample

The sample consists of 300 participants with a stuck of 75.30 % females. The mean age was 49 years (min. = 18 years, max. = 72 years). The sample contained 67 % employees, 14.30 % executives, 15.30 % self-employed, 1.30 % pensioners and 2.1 % unemployment persons. 27.70 % participants reported a work experience of 2–5 years, 14 % participants reported 6–10 years, 25.70 % participants reported 11–20 years and 32.70 % participants reported 21 or more years. The biggest part was allied: 41.30 % participants reported to be married, 33.70 % reported to be in a relationship. 15.30 % participants reported to be single and 9 % divorced. .70 % participants reported to be widowed. 46.70 % participants stated to have one child at least. Acquisition was carried out via internet.

3.8.2.2 Instruments

Art-of-Living Questionnaire

For the art-of-living-questionnaire see, Chap. 2. We selected five components of the art of living, namely openness, self-efficacy, self-determined way of living, self-knowledge and optimization. Our main selection criterion was relevance for the construct art-of-living with respect to the construct self-fulfillment in working life.

Measuring Self-Fulfillment in Working Life

According to Müller (2003), components of self-fulfillment in working life are vocational self-efficacy, self-worth management, self-promotion and self-motivation.

Self-efficacy was measured by the *vocational self-efficacy-scale* (Abele et al. 2000). The six-item instrument shows a Cronbach's α of .73, for the present study resulted $\alpha = .76$. An example item is *I know exactly that I can meet the requirements of my profession if I just want to*. The subjects specify their agreement to the items by a 6-pointed Likert-scale ranging from *strongly disagree* to *strongly agree*.

Self-worth management was measured with the *organizational-self-worth-scale* of Kanning and Schnitker (2004). For the internal consistency (Cronbach's α) they found values ranging from .86 to .96 in seven different samples. In the present study resulted .95. For responding to the items there is a 6-pointed Likert-scale available (from *strongly disagree* to *strongly agree*). An example item is *One takes me seriously*.

The measurement of self-promotion was realized by the homonymous four-item subscale of the *Impression Management Scale* (Bolino and Turnley 1999). An example item is *I speak with pride about my experience or education*. The 5-pointed Likert-scale ranges from *never behave this way* to *often behave this way*. Cronbach's α was found to be .78. In the present study this value was replicated ($\alpha = .80$).

For measurement the self-motivation we selected two scales of the *Questionnaire for self-leadership* (Butzmann 2011): the scale *behavioral focus* ($\alpha = .72$) as well as *natural reward focus* ($\alpha = .78$). The 6-pointed Likert scale ranges from *strongly disagree* to *strongly agree*. An example item for the first mentioned scale is *I give my work a pleasant ambience*, for the second mentioned *At work I always find something that makes me happy*.

Measuring Subjective Occupational Success

To capture the construct self-fulfillment in working life as accurately as possible, we added components of *subjective occupational success*. In this study, we consider *career satisfaction, success compared with colleagues, vocational identity,* and *global job satisfaction* as these components.

The measurement of career satisfaction was realized by the *Questionnaire for career satisfaction* of Greenhaus et al. (1990), which shows an internal consistency (Cronbach's α) of .88. In the present study resulted .90. An example item is *I'm satisfied with the success that I have achieved in my career so far*. The consent of the subjects to the items was recorded by a 6-pointed Likert-scale ranging from *strongly disagree* to *strongly agree*.

To determine the subjective success compared with colleagues it was used a single item according to Dette (2005): *If you compare yourself with your former student / education colleagues, how successful do you rate your current professional development?* It was used a 6-pointed Likert scale ranging from *strongly disagree* to *strongly agree*.

The vocational identity was captured by the three-item scale *job involvement* of the *Involvement Scale* according to Moser and Schuler (1993) with a 7-pointed Likert-scale (from *strongly agree* to *strongly disagree*). An example item is *The work means to me a lot more than just money*. Moser and Schuster found the Cronbach's α to be .64, in the present study was found a value of .79.

The global job satisfaction was asked by a single item (*Everything considered together: Are you satisfied with your current job on the whole?*). The subjects specified their agreement using a six-pointed Kunin-scale ranging from the view of a sad face to the view of a happy face [see Nerdinger et al. (2011)].

3.8.3 Results

3.8.3.1 Relationship Between Art-of-Living and Self-Fulfillment in Working Life

The correlation of the total art-of-living score and the total score of the self-fulfillment in working life amounted to .65. Table 3.11 gives an overview about the correlations based on the subscales.

Table 3.11 Correlations of art-of-living and self-fulfillment in working life on the level of subscales

Art-of-living	Self-fulfillment in working life			
	Vocational self-efficacy	Self-worth management	Self-promotion	Self-motivation
Openness	.47***	.38***	.25***	.40***
Self-efficacy	.66***	.42***	.23***	.46***
Self-determined way of living	.63***	.52***	.23***	.57***
Self-knowledge	.48***	.32***	.11	.36***
Optimization	.57***	.33***	.13*	.40***

$N = 300$
*** $p < .01$; * $p < .05$

Table 3.12 Correlations of art-of-living with subjective occupational success on the level of subscales

Art-of-living	Subjective occupational success			
	Career satisfaction	Vocational identity	Global job satisfaction	Success comp. w. colleagues
Openness	.33***	.41***	.28***	.40***
Self-efficacy	.49***	.36***	.30***	.45***
Self-determined way of living	.58***	.54***	.50***	.48***
Self-knowledge	.33***	.26***	.18**	.25***
Optimization	.42***	.26***	.25***	.36***

Success comp. w. colleagues success compared with colleagues
$N = 300$
*** $p < .01$; ** $p < .01$

To determine the predictive usefulness of the art-of-living variables we calculated a regression analysis. The art-of-living subscales were used to predict the self-fulfillment in working life total score.[2] The explained variance amounted to 56 %. Significance turned out for three of the five predictors, namely *openness* ($\beta = .14$), *self-efficacy* ($\beta = .18$) and *self-determined way of living* ($\beta = .48$). From this results, we conclude that art-of-living allows the prediction of self-fulfillment in working life.

Relationship Between Art-of-Living and the Components of Subjective Occupational Success

All art-of-living subscales as well as the total art-of-living score showed significant positive relationships with the components of the subjective occupational success. The highest correlation of the art-of-living full scale was found for career satisfaction (.53), the lowest for global job satisfaction (.38). For vocational identity was found .46, for success compared with colleagues .49. The correlations on level of the subscales are shown in Table 3.12.

3.8.4 Discussion

We used art-of-living scales to predict variables of working life. In a sample of 300 people we could show that art-of-living shows systematic relationships to

[2]Because the component self-promotion of subjective occupational success showed rather low correlations ($r < .30$) with the subscales of self-fulfillment in working life, it was assumed that it isn't an adequate indicator for the targeting construct and excluded from the regression analyzes.

self-fulfillment in working life and subjective occupational success. *Self-determined way of living* shows high correlations to all self-fulfillment variables and the highest to subjective occupational success. Although one cannot derive causal mechanisms from these correlations it is justified to try to enhance these art-of-living variables in order to influence occupational success.

3.9 Summary

Bernhard Schmitz

The aim of this chapter was to continue the validation of the art-of-living questionnaire. We proceeded as follows. First, we tried to show that art-of-living is related to its goal the attainment of well-being. Therefore we used different measures of well-being, the satisfaction with life scale (SWLS), the subjective happiness scale (SHS), the authentic happiness inventory (AHI), psychological well-being (PWB) and eudaimonic well-being (EWB) and depression (BDI). Second, we investigated the relationship between art-of-living and flourishing which could be regarded even as a more appropriate criterion. In the third step we studied the relationship between personality measured by the Big Five and art-of-living. The main question was whether art-of-living could be determined mainly by personality. Then we studied the similarity between other main ways for leading a good life and art-of-living, strengths and virtues and orientations to happiness. A further step in validation was the analyses of the relationship between other important constructs of positive psychology resilience, sense of coherence, self-regulation and wisdom. In addition, we investigated the relations to anxiety, mindfulness and emotional intelligence. Following this more content oriented validation we tried a more methodological way of validation in that we applied other measures for art-of-living in addition to the questionnaire. One additional measure was the peer estimation of art-of-living and the other instrument was a situational judgement test (SJT) of art-of-living. Finally we looked at relationships between art-of-living and work-related variables.

The correlation to the most of the criterion measures of well-being was high (.59 for SWLS, .62 for SHS and .69 for AHI, for the PWB mean of the 6 measures .57 and to EWB .38). For depression (BDI) resulted -.57, for anxiety -.75.

The multiple regression with SWLS as criterion and art-of-living as predictor yielded in a sample of 1105 subjects a multiple $R = .78$ and a $R^2 = .61$ ($p < .001$)

The correlations to flourishing were highest to the Seligman's PERMA measure (.76).

Regarding personality the correlations between art-of-living and the Big Five were between .21 and −.59 showing that the art-of-living can be predicted by personality. The multiple regression proved that well-being (SWLS) could be predicted by personality but art-of-living could add a significant and remarkable part for the prediction above personality. For the analyses of communalities between strengths and virtues and art-of-living revealed all significant correlations and the highest correlations to transcendence and wisdom. A similar conclusion than for personality holds, there are communalities between art-of-living and strengths and virtues but art-of-living has more to offer than the strengths and virtues short form. With respect to OTH the art-of-living-strategies are significantly related to all orientations that means they provide strategies related to all the three orientations with a little higher relationship to engagement although no direct measure of engagement or flow is included in the art-of-living.

Measures of important constructs of Positive Psychology like resilience, sense of coherence and wisdom as well as minflulness and emotional intelligence yield also high correlations to art-of-living but it could be shown that art-of-living adds to each of these constructs to predict well-being. We also tried to develop another measure of art-of-living using a situational judgement test (SJT), which showed encouraging results with respect to its consistency and its correlation with the self-report questionnaire.

The correspondence with peer ratings reveals correlations which have a comparable magnitude than for similar measures, e.g. the self-peer correlation for SHS yielded a mean $r = .54$ (cf. Lyubomirsky and Lepper 1999) (for the SWLS s. Pavot and Diener 1993) although happiness can much easier be observed than strategies like balance.

In the study analyzing the relationships between work related variables like subjective occupational success and self-fulfillment in working life we found meaningful correlations, allowing the interpretation that art-of-living is also important for working life. Therefore, in the intervention chapter we also try to enhance art-of-living with the goal to enhance happiness in the working context.

In sum, we found high correlations with similar constructs like strengths and virtues and wisdom (convergent validity). There were low or no relationships with different constructs (social desirability) (divergent validity). We could show that art-of-living has high relationships with criteria like different forms of well-being or flourishing. We could show that art-of-living adds to the prediction of well-being in addition to personality (Big Five) (incremental validity). Further we could demonstrate that ratings of art-of-living of self and peers covary and that an overall scale for art-of-living can also be measured by a SJT. Taken together, there were clear hints that the validation process of art-of-living has left its primary phase.

References

Abele, A. E., Spurk, D., & Volmer, J. (2011). The construct of career success: Measurement issues and an empirical example. *Zeitschrift für Arbeitsmarktforschung, 43*(3), 195–206.

Abele, A. E., Stief, M., & Andrä, M. S. (2000). Zur ökonomischen Erfassung beruflicher Selbstwirksamkeitserwartungen-Neukonstruktion einer BSW-Skala. *Zeitschrift für Arbeits-und Organisationspsychologie, 44*(3), 145–151.

Amelang, M., Bartussek, D., Stemmler, G., & Hagemann, D. (2006). *Differentielle Psychologie und Persönlichkeitsforschung* (6. Auflage). Stuttgart: W. Kohlhammer.

Antonovsky, A. (1987). *Unraveling the mystery of health: How people manage stress and stay well.* San Francisco: Jossey Bass.

Ardelt, M. (2003). Empirical assessment of a three-dimensional wisdom scale. *Research on Aging, 25*(3), 275–324.

Ardelt, M. (2006). *3-dimensionale Weisheitsskala*. Retrieved May 31, 2011 from http://www.geo.de/GEO/interaktiv/tests/50033.html

Baer, R. A., Smith, G. T., & Allen, K. B. (2004). Assessment of mindfulness by self-report. The Kentucky inventory of mindfulness skills. *Assessment, 11*(3), 191–206.

Baltes, P. B., & Kunzmann, U. (2003). Wisdom. *The Psychologist*, 131–133.

Baltes, P. B., & Smith, J. (1990). Toward a psychology of wisdom and its ontogenesis. In R. Sternberg (Ed.), *Wisdom: Its nature, origins, and development* (pp. 87–120). Cambridge: Cambridge University Press.

Baltes, P. B., & Smith, J. (2008). The fascination of wisdom: Its nature, ontogeny, and function. *Perspectives on Psychological Science, 3*(1), 56–64.

Baltes, P. B., & Staudinger, U. M. (1993). The search for psychology of wisdom. *Current Directions in Psychological Science, 2*(3), 75–80.

Baltes, P., Staudinger, U. M., Maercker, A., & Smith, J. (1995). People nominated as wise: A comparative study of wisdom-related knowledge. *Psychology and Aging*, 155–166.

Bandura, A. (1977). Self-efficacy: Toward a unifying theory of behavioral change. *Psychological Review, 84*(2), 191.

Beck, A. T., Ward, C., & Mendelson, M. (1961). Beck depression inventory (BDI). *Archives of General Psychiatry, 4*(6), 561–571.

Beck, A. T., Steer, R. A., & Brown, G. K. (1996). *Manual for the Beck depression inventory-II*. San Antonio: Psychological Corporation.

Bellhäuser, H., Roth, A., & Schmitz, B. (2015). SRL@U: Validierung des Fragebogens zur Erhebung des selbstregulierten Lernens an der Universität. Vortrag auf der 3. Tagung der Gesellschaft für empirische Bildungsforschung (GEBF) in Bochum, 11.-13.03.2015.

Bending, B. (2013). *Fragebogen zur Erfassung der Lebenskunst mittels Situational Judgement Test und die Zusammenhänge zu Wohlbefinden* (Bachelor thesis). Technische Universität Darmstadt.

Bengel, J., Strittmatter, R., & Willmann, H. (2001). *Was erhält Menschen gesund? Antonovskys Modell der Salutogenese—Diskussionsstand und Stellenwert*. Köln: Bundeszentrale für gesundheitliche Aufklärung.

Berg, J. M., Dutton, J. E., & Wrzesniewski, A. (2013). Job crafting and meaningful work. In B. J. Dik, Z. S. Byrne & M. F. Steger (Eds.), *Purpose and meaning in the workplace* (pp. 81–104). Washington, DC: American Psychological Association.

Bierhoff, H. W., & Herner, M. J. (2003). Selbstüberzeugung. In G. F. Müller (Ed.), *Selbstverwirklichung im Arbeitsleben* (pp. 85–104). Lengerich: Pabst Science.

Bledow, R., & Frese, M. (2009). A situational jugement test of personal initiative and its relationship to performance. *Personnel Psychology, 62*(2), 229–258.

Bolino, M. C., & Turnley, W. H. (1999). Measuring impression management in organizations: A scale development based on the Jones and Pittman taxonomy. *Organizational Research Methods, 2*(2), 187–206.

Borkenau, P., Friedel, A., & Wolfradt, U. (2011). Standardisierte Persönlichkeitsfragebögen. In L. F. Hornke, M. Amelang & M. Kersting (Hrsg.), Persönlichkeitsdiagnostik (Enzyklopädie der Psychologie, Bd. 4, S. 1-72).

Bozeman, D. P., & Kacmar, K. M. (1997). A cybernetic model of impression management processes in organizations. *Organizational Behavior and Human Decision Processes, 69*(1), 9–30.

Brand, H. (2003). Selbstpräsentation im Arbeitsleben. In G. F. Müller (Ed.), *Selbstverwirklichung im Arbeitsleben* (pp. 105–122). Lengerich: Pabst Science.

Buschor, C., Proyer, R. T., & Ruch, W. (2013). Self-and peer-rated character strengths: How do they relate to satisfaction with life and orientations to happiness? *The Journal of Positive Psychology, 8*(2), 116–127.

Butzmann, B. (2011). *Eignungs-und kompetenzspezifische Bedingungen und Erfolgsindikatoren von Führung durch Selbstführung* (Univ. diss.). Koblenz, Landau (Pfalz), Univ.

Costa, P. T., & McCrae, R. R. (1992a). Normal personality assessment in clinical practice: The NEO Personality Inventory. *Psychological Assessment, 4*(1), 5.

Costa, P. T., Jr., & McCrae, R. R. (1992b). *Revised NEO personality inventory (NEO-PI-R) and NEO five-factor inventory (NEO-FFI) professional manual*. Odessa, FL: Psychological Assessment Resources.

Csikszentmihalyi, M. (1990). *Flow: The Psychology of Optimal Experience*. New York: HarperCollins.

Dette, D. E. (2005). *Berufserfolg und Lebenszufriedenheit*. Eine längsschnittliche Analyse der Zusammenhänge.

Dette, D. E., Abele, A. E., & Renner, O. (2004). Zur Definition und Messung von Berufserfolg: Theoretische Überlegungen und metaanalytische Befunde zum Zusammenhang von externen und internen Laufbahnerfolgsmaßen. *Zeitschrift für Personalpsychologie, 3*(4), 170–183.

Diener, E. D., Emmons, R. A., Larsen, R. J., & Griffin, S. (1985). The satisfaction with life scale. *Journal of Personality Assessment, 49*(1), 71–75.

Diener, E., Wirtz, D., Tov, W., Kim-Prieto, C., Choi, D. W., Oishi, S., et al. (2010). New well-being measures: Short scales to assess flourishing and positive and negative feelings. *Social Indicators Research, 97*(2), 143–156.

Fliege, H., Rose, M., Arck, P., Levenstein, S., & Klapp, B. F. (2001). Validierung des „Perceived Stress Questionnaire" (PSQ) an einer deutschen Stichprobe. *Diagnostica, 47*(3), 142–152.

Fröhlich-Gildhoff, K., & Rönnau-Böse, M. (2009). *Resilienz*. München: Reinhardt.

Funder, D. C., & Colvin, C. R. (1988). Friends and strangers: acquaintanceship, agreement, and the accuracy of personality judgment. *Journal of Personality and Social Psychology, 55*(1), 149–158.

Funder, D. C., & Dobroth, K. M. (1987). Differences between traits: Properties associated with interjudge agreement. *Journal of Personality and Social Psychology, 52*(2), 409.

Furnham, A., & Lester, D. (2012). The development of a short measure of character strength. *European Journal of Psychological Assessment, 28*(2), 95–101.

Goldberg, L. R. (1981). Language and individual differences: The search for universals in personality Lexicons. *Review of Personality and Social Psychology, 2*(1), 141–165.

Grant, A. M. (2007). Relational job design and the motivation to make a prosocial difference. *Academy of Management Review, 32*(2), 393–417.

Greenhaus, J. H., Parasuraman, S., & Wormley, W. M. (1990). Effects of race on organizational experiences, job performance evaluations, and career outcomes. *Academy of Management Journal, 33*(1), 64–86.

Hackman, J. R., & Oldham, G. R. (1980). *Work Redesign*. Reading, MA: Addison-Wesley.

Hayes, S. C., Strosahl, K., Wilson, K. G., & Bissett, R. T. (2004). Measuring experiential avoidance: A preliminary test of a working model. *The Psychological Record, 54*(4), 553.

Heidenreich, T., & Michalak, J. (2006). Achtsamkeit und Akzeptanz als Prinzipien in der Psychotherapie. *PiD-Psychotherapie im Dialog, 7*(3), 235–240.

Herzberg, F., Mausner, B., & Snyderman, B. B. (1959). *The motivation to work*. New York: John Wiley & Sons.

Hone, L. C., Jarden, A., Schofield, G. M., & Duncan, S. (2014). Measuring flourishing: The impact of operational definitions on the prevalence of high levels of well-being. *International Journal of Well-being, 4*(1), 62–90.

Huppert, F. A., & So, T. T. (2013). Flourishing across Europe: Application of a new conceptual framework for defining well-being. *Social Indicators Research, 110*(3), 837–861.

Huppertz, M. (2003). Die Bedeutung des Zen-Buddhismus für die Dialektisch-Behaviorale Therapie. *PPmP-Psychotherapie· Psychosomatik· Medizinische Psychologie, 53*(9/10), 376–383.

John, O. P., & Srivastava, S. (1999). The Big-Five trait taxonomy: History, measurement, and theoretical perspectives. In L. A. Pervin & O. P. John (Eds.), Handbook of personality: Theory and research (Vol. 2, pp. 102–138). New York: Guilford Press.

Judge, T. A., Higgins, C. A., Thoresen, C. J., & Barrick, M. R. (1999). The big five personality traits, general mental ability, and career success across the life span. *Personnel Psychology, 52*(3), 621–652.

Kabat-Zinn, J. (2003). Mindfulness-based interventions in context: Past, present, and future. *Clinical Psychology: Science and Practice, 10*(2), 144–156.

Kanning, U. P. (2003). Selbstwertmanagement. In G. F. Müller (Ed.), *Selbstverwirklichung im Arbeitsleben* (pp. 59–84). Lengerich: Pabst Science.

Kanning, U. P., & Schnitker, R. (2004). Übersetzung und Validierung einer Skala zur Messung des organisationsbezogenen Selbstwertes. *Zeitschrift für Personalpsychologie, 3*(3), 112–121.

Kekes, J. (1988). *The examined life*. Cranbury, NJ: Associated University Press.

Kelava, A., & Moosbrugger, H. (2012). Deskriptivstatistische Evaluation von Items (Itemanalyse) und Testwertverteilungen. In H. Moosbrugger & A. Kelava (Hrsg.), Testtheorie und Fragebogenkonstruktion (pp. 75–102). Berlin: Springer.

Keyes, C. L. (2002). The mental health continuum: From languishing to flourishing in life. *Journal of Health and Social Behavior, 43*(2), 207–222.

Klimek, N. (2015). *Validierung von Fragebögen zu Flourishing und der Zusammenhang mit Lebenskunst.* (Unpublished Master's thesis, Technical Universitity of Darmstadt, Germany).

Knoll, N., Scholz, U., & Rieckmann, N. (2011). *Einführung Gesundheitspsychologie*. München: Ernst Reinhardt Verlag.

Krankenhagen, M. E. (2015). *Mehr oder weniger ein Lebenskünstler—Eine Studie über das Konstrukt Lebenskunst und dessen Erhebung mittels Situational Judgement Test* (Unpublished Masters' thesis). Technical University of Darmstadt, Germany.

Lautz, A. (2013). *Art-of-living and personality, well-being and depression* (Unpublished bachelor's thesis). Technical University of Darmstadt, Germany.

Lounsbury, J. W., Loveland, J. M., Sundstrom, E. D., Gibson, L. W., Drost, A. W., & Hamrick, F. L. (2003). An investigation of personality traits in relation to career satisfaction. *Journal of Career Assessment, 11*(3), 287–307.

Lyubomirsky, S. (2008). *The how of happiness: A scientific approach to getting the life you want*. New York: Penguin.

Lyubomirsky, S., & Lepper, H. S. (1999). A measure of subjective happiness: Preliminary reliability and construct validation. *Social Indicators Research, 46*, 137–155.

Maxwell, N. (2004). In defense of seeking wisdom. *Metaphilosophy, 35*(5), 733–743.

McCrae, R. R., & Costa, P. T., Jr. (1999). A five-factor theory of personality. *Handbook of Personality: Theory and Research, 2*, 139–153.

Mertel, B. (2006). *Arbeitszufriedenheit–eine empirische Studie zu Diagnose, Erfassung und Modifikation in einem führenden Unternehmen des Automotives*. Retrieved August 31, 2016 from http://d-nb.info/981263240/34

Mieg, H. A., & Woschnak, U. (2002). Die berufliche Identität von Umweltdienstleistern. Altes, neues oder ohne Berufsbild? *Arbeit, 11*(3), 185–198.

Moser, K., & Schuler, H. (1993). Validität einer deutschsprachigen Involvement-Skala. *Zeitschrift für Differentielle und diagnostische Psychologie, 14*(1), 27–36.

Müller, G. F. (2003). *Selbstverwirklichung im Arbeitsleben*. Lengerich: Pabst Science.

Nafziger, R. (2001). *Der Primat der Solidarität.: Impulse für eine weltorientierte Gesellschaft, Politik und Wirtschaft*. Norderstedt: Books on Demand GmbH (elektronische version).

Nerdinger, F. W., Blickle, G., & Schaper, N. (2011). *Arbeits-und Organisationspsychologie (Lehrbuch mit Online-Materialien)*. Berlin: Springer.

Paunonen, S. V., & Oneill, T. A. (2010). Self-reports, peer rating and construct validity. *European Journal of Personality, 24*(3), 189–206.

Pavot, W., & Diener, E. (1993). Review of the satisfaction with life scale. *Psychological Assessment, 5*(2), 164.

Peterson, C., & Seligman, M. E. (2004). *Character strengths and virtues: A handbook and classification*. Oxford: Oxford University Press.

Peterson, C., Park, N., & Seligman, M. E. (2005). Orientations to happiness and life satisfaction: The full life versus the empty life. *Journal of Happiness Studies, 6*(1), 25–41.

Radloff, L. S. (1977). The CES-D scale a self-report depression scale for research in the general population. *Applied Psychological Measurement, 1*(3), 385–401.

Rammstedt, B., & John, O. P. (2007). Measuring personality in one minute or less: A 10-item short version of the Big Five Inventory in English and German. *Journal of Research in Personality, 41*(1), 203–212.

Rindermann, H. (2009). *Emotionale-Kompetenz-Fragebogen (EKF) Manual*. Göttingen: Hogrefe.

Ruch, W., Proyer, R. T., Harzer, C., & Park, N. P. (2010). Ways to Happiness in German-speaking countries: The adaption of the German version of the Orientatinos of Happiness Questionaire in paper-pencil and internet samples. *European Journal of Psychology Assessment, 26*(3), 227–234.

Rupp, C. (2014). *Lebenskunst—Erfassung des Konstrukts mittels Situational Judgement Test* [*Art of living—Measuring the construct with a SJT*]. (Unpublished Bachelors' Thesis). Technical University of Darmstadt, Germany.

Ryan, R. M., & Deci, E. L. (2001). On happiness and human potentials: A review of research on hedonic and eudaimonic well-being. *Annual Review of Psychology, 52*(1), 141–166.

Ryff, C. D. (1989). Happiness is everything, or is it? Explorations on the meaning of psychological well-being. *Journal of Personality and Social Psychology, 57*(6), 1069.

Ryff, C. D., & Keyes, C. L. M. (1995). The structure of psychological well-being revisited. *Journal of Personality and Social Psychology, 69*(4), 719.

Schahn, J., & Amelang, M. (1992). *Mittelwertsunterschiede zwischen Selbst- und Fremdbeurteilungen: Eine vernachlässigte Größe? Diagnostica, 38*(3), 187–208.

Schiffrin, H. H., & Nelson, S. K. (2010). Stressed and happy? Investigating the relationship between happiness and perceived stress. *Journal of Happiness Studies, 11*(1), 33–39.

Schmid, W. (2004). *Mit sich befreundet sein*. Von der Lebenskunst im Umgang mit sich selbst: Suhrkamp Verlag.

Schmitz, B., & Schmidt, A. (2014). Development of a questionnaire measuring the art of living. *Psychologie in Erziehung und Unterricht, 61*(4), 252–266.

Schmitz, B., & Wiese, B. S. (2006). New perspectives for the evaluation of training sessions in self-regulated learning: Time-series analyses of diary data. *Contemporary Educational Psychology, 31*(1), 64–96.

Schröder, T. & König, P. (2014) *Optimierung des Fragebogens zur Lebenskunst durch Hinzufügen von zusätzlichen Skalen*. Bachelor thesis. Gutachter: Prof. Dr. Bernhard Schmitz, Dipl Psych Sylvana Keller.

Schumacher, B. (2015). *Zusammenhang von Lebenskunst und Charakterstärken und Einfluss auf Lebenszufriedenheit und Wohlbefinden*. (Unpublished Masters' thesis). Technical University of Darmstadt, Germany.

Schumacher, J., Leppert, K., Gunzelmann, T., Strauß, B., & Brähler, E. (2004). *Resilienzskala RS-25 und Kurzform RS-11*. © Schumacher: Leppert, Gunzelmann, Strauß & Brähler, Unversitäten Jena und Leipzig.

Schumacher, J., Wilz, G., Gunzelmann, T., & Brähler, E. (2000). Die sense of coherence scale von Antonovsky. *PPmP-Psychotherapie· Psychosomatik· Medizinische Psychologie, 50*(12), 472–482.

Seligman, M. E. (1995). *Learned helplessness: A theory for the age of personal control*. Oxford: University Press.

Seligman, M. E. (2011). *P*. How to change your mind and your life. Vintage: Learned optimism.

Seligman, M. E. P. (2002). *Authentic happiness*. New York: Free Press.

Seligman, M. E., Steen, T. A., Park, N., & Peterson, C. (2005). Positive psychology progress: Empirical validation of interventions. *American Psychologist, 60*(5), 410.

Sin, N., & Lyubomirsky, S. (2009). *Enhancing well-being and alleviating depressive symptoms* with positive psychology interventions: A practice-friendly meta-analysis. *Journal of Clinical Psychology, 65*(5), 467–487.

Spinath, F. (2000). Validität von Fremdbeurteilungen: Einflussfaktoren auf die Konvergenz von Selbst- und Fremdeinschätzungen in Persönlichkeitseinschätzungen. In Sarris, V., Amelang, M., Birbaumer, N., Strack, F., & Wilkening, F. (Hrsg.). Psychologia Universalis, Neue Reihe, Band 20. Lengerich: Pabst.

Staudinger, U. M., Smith, J., & Baltes, P. B. (1992). Wisdom-related knowledge in a life review task: Age differences and the role of professional specialization. *Psychology and Aging, 7*, 271–281.

Sternberg, R. J. (1998). A balance theory of wisdom. *Review of General Psychology, 2*(4), 347.

Stief, M. (2001). *Selbstwirksamkeitserwartungen, Ziele und Berufserfolg: Eine Längsschnittstudie*. Aachen: Shaker.

Ströhle, G., Nachtigall, C., Michalak, J., & Heidenreich, T. (2010). Die Erfassung von Achtsamkeit als mehrdimensionales Konstrukt. Die deutsche Version des Kentucky Inventory of Mindfulness Skills (KIMS-D). *Zeitschrift für Klinische Psychologie und Psychotherapie, 39*(1), 1–12.

Thiele, L. P. (2006). *The heart of judgment practical wisdom, neuroscience, and narrative*. Cambridge: Cambridge University Press.

Treichel, K. (2015). *A German version of the questionnaire for eudamonic well-being* (Unpublished bachelor's thesis). Technische Universität Darmstadt, Darmstadt, Germany.

Wagnild, G., & Young, H. (1993). Development and psychometric. *Journal of Nursing Measurement, 1*(2), 165–178.

Waterman, A. S., Schwartz, S. J., Zamboanga, B. L., Ravert, R. D., Williams, M. K., Bede Agocha, V., et al. (2010). The questionnaire for eudaimonic well-being: Psychometric properties, demographic comparisons, and evidence of validity. *The Journal of Positive Psychology, 5*(1), 41–61.

Watson, D., & Clark, L. A. (1991). Self- versus peer ratings of specific emotional traits: Evidence of convergent and discriminant validity. *Journal of Personality and Social Psychology, 60*(6), 927–940.

Weber, H., & Rammsayer, T. (2012). *Differentielle Psychologie- Persönlichkeitsforschung* Göttingen: Hogrefe. Aberufen von Google Books. Zugriff am December 11, 2014 unter: http://books.google.de/books?id=v9HSzamG0M8C&pg=PA42&lpg=PA42&dq=methode.

Werner, E. (1993). Risk, resilience, and recovery: Perspectives from the Kauai Longitudinal Study. *Development and Psychopathology, 5*, 503–515.

Wrzesniewski, A., McCauley, C., Rozin, P., & Schwartz, B. (1997). Jobs, careers, and callings: People‘s relations to their work. *Journal of Research in Personality, 31*, 21–33.

Zimmerman, B. J. (2000). Attaining self-regulation: A social cognitive perspective. In M. Boekaerts, P. R. Pintrich & M, Zeidner (Eds.), *Handbook of self-regulation* (pp. 13–39). San Diego: Academic Press.

Chapter 4
Measurement of Art-of-Living in Daily Life by Diaries

4.1 Introduction

Alexander Stahlmann, Bernhard Schmitz

As we showed in the preliminary chapters, art-of-living comprises a theoretically well-grounded construct that can be assessed both reliably and validly by the art-of-living questionnaire. Furthermore, art-of-living is strongly related to well-being, physical health and psychological flourishing. However, so far, we merely focused on cross-sectional analyses, neglecting individual trajectories in art-of-living. Moreover, the precise relational pattern between art-of-living and well-being is still unclear.

In this chapter, we will address these issues by introducing process analyses as a method to estimate short-term changes in individual art-of-living patterns. For this purpose, we conducted a broad diary study and assessed individual trajectories in art-of-living over the course of 28 consecutive days. In addition, we related the daily measures to the established cross-sectional questionnaire in a comprehensive pretest and posttest framework.

Gradually, we will approach the question whether art-of-living and well-being are branched in a causal framework and discuss potentially temporal antecedents of a high level in well-being. At first, as a premise, we will evaluate validity and stability of overall art-of-living as well as the particular subscales by matching the process data with the results from the pretest and posttest protocol. By this means, we aspire to gain a better understanding whether the construct describes a stable, temporally consistent trait variable or an unstable, temporally inconsistent state variable. Subsequently, we will address the temporal interaction of art-of-living and situational factors, that is, current important events either perceived as positively connoted uplifts or negatively connoted hassles. As contemporaneous research showed, current events comprise significant predictors of well-being and physical health. Consequently, we will evaluate if these effects can be replicated with respect

B. Schmitz, *Art-of-Living*, Social Indicators Research Series 63,
DOI 10.1007/978-3-319-45324-8_4

to art-of-living. Thereafter, we will investigate the relational pattern between art-of-living and well-being by evaluating both synchronous and asynchronous temporal correlations. We will discuss hints regarding causation and introduce process dynamics as a promising predictor of a high level in well-being. We will summarize our results in a comprehensive overall discussion and provide suggestions regarding prospective research.

4.2 Method

Alexander Stahlmann, Bernhard Schmitz

4.2.1 *Sample*

The sample consisted of $N = 53$ participants (♀ = 73.60 %) who were mainly recruited from a German university ($n = 92.50$ %). Most of the participants reported German as their native descent ($n = 90.60$ %), and the mean age was $M = 23.90$ year ($SD = 3.78$ years). Every participant who completed the pretest and posttest automatically entered an overall prize competition awarded with 20€, 30€, or 50€ raffled at the end of the study. All participants completed either pretest or posttest and supplied at least 75 % of the diaries. Missing values were handled by an expectation maximization algorithm provided by Honaker et al. (2011). By this means, data for 5 of 53 pretest and posttest submissions (9.43 %) and for 168 of 1484 diaries (11.32 %) was imputed.

4.2.2 *Procedure*

Framed by a comprehensive pretest and posttest protocol to assess overall art-of-living and well-being, all participants supplied diaries over the course of 28 consecutive days. The diary was derived directly from the instruments utilized in the pretest and the posttest, augmented with short measures of affect and current important events. Every instrument except open questions was scaled on a seven-point Likert scale ranging from 1 = "strongly disagree" to 7 = "strongly agree". All measures were completely computer-based and could be transmitted via home computer or mobile phone.

4.2.3 *Instruments*

4.2.3.1 Pretest and Posttest

Pretest and posttest were composed of the art-of-living questionnaire (AoL; cf. Chap. 2) as well as the satisfaction with life scale (SWLS; Diener et al. 1985) in the

German localization by Glaesmer et al. (2011). As noted by the authors, the SWLS is specifically concerned with cognitive components of well-being. The German version of the SWLS accords with general demands of psychometrics with an internal consistency of $\alpha = .92$ and item-total correlations $r > .70$ and was validated with both convergent and discriminant scales. Exclusively in the pretest, demographics (i.e. gender, profession, nationality and gender) were assessed.

4.2.3.2 Diary

For the diary the art-of-living questionnaire was condensed in a representative selection of 25 items regarding 13 of the foremost 14 subscales. The subscale "integrating different areas of life" was intentionally dropped because we questioned the daily relevance. The subscale "shaping of living conditions" was measured by one characteristic item while the remaining subscales were represented by two typical items each. With respect to overall art-of-living, an aggregated score was estimated by averaging the respective subscale signatures.

To assess well-being, we presented all five items of the SWLS in the German localization (Glaesmer et al. 2011) and four representative items regarding positive and negative affect (PANAS, Watson et al. 1988) translated by Krohne et al. (1996). Just as the SWLS, the positive and negative affect schedule satisfies current expectations in psychometrics with an internal consistency of $\alpha > .85$ and was validated with measures of personality, vigilance and anxiety.

To address present states rather than stable traits in art-of-living and well-being, we supplemented the usual item wording with the temporal cue "today" and changed the tense from simple present to simple past (e.g. "Today, I managed to overcome disruptions by direct actions" or "Today, I was satisfied with my life").

Complementing the short-version of the art-of-living questionnaire, the amount of applied art-of-living-related coping-strategies was assessed via open question. Regarding the statistical analyses, we simply cumulated the total count of mentioned strategies on a daily base.

Current important events were addressed by open questions. By this means, participants were prompted to mention and rate their daily experiences with respect to the perceived importance of the event. Concerning the statistical analyses, we distinguished positive events (uplifts) from negative events (hassles) and computed the total amount as well as the mean relative importance of the respective event categories, thus obtaining four discriminative estimators for each day.

4.2.4 Psychometric Properties of the Diary

As 53 participants supplied 28 diaries, the psychometric evaluation of the diary was based on $N = 1484$ observations. Overall mean level statistics, Cronbach's α, item-total correlations and split-half reliability are depicted in Table 4.1.

Table 4.1 Psychometric properties of the diary: mean level scores, Cronbach's α, split-half reliability and item-total correlations of the respective subscale with overall art-of-living

Scale	Mean level	Cronbach's α	Item-total correlation	Split-half reliability
Coping	4.68	.75	.71	.90
Openness	4.54	.52	.68	.84
Self-determined way of living	5.22	.74	.82	.86
Savoring	5.07	.78	.60	.84
Serenity	4.58	.76	.67	.85
Balance	4.89	.60	.79	.84
Social contact	5.23	.77	.58	.79
Self-knowledge	5.53	.64	.67	.95
Shaping of living conditions	4.52	a)	.60	.87
Physical care	4.33	.79	.58	.65
Optimization	5.24	.77	.66	.85
Self-efficacy	4.73	.75	.69	.87
Positive attitude towards life	5.10	.88	.79	.89
Overall art-of-living	4.90	.92	–	.96
SWLS	4.67	.90	–	.87
PANAS—positive affect	4.75	.64	–	.91
PANAS—negative affect	3.11	.80	–	.88

Explanatory note (a) The subscale "shaping of living conditions" consists of only one item. Therefore, for this scale, Cronbach's alpha coefficient could not be computed

Mean level scores for a particular scale or subscale were computed by taking the average of every respective observation. With respect to art-of-living, the subscales ranged between $Min = 4.33$ and $Max = 5.53$, evening out at the overall art-of-living $Mean = 4.90$ with $SD = .36$. Thus, the mean statistics generally accord with the psychometrics of the art-of-living questionnaire reported in Chap. 2. On the whole, the mean level of the SWLS ($Mean = 4.67$) aligns with the score reported by the authors ($Mean = 4.98$). As we scaled the positive and negative affect schedule on a seven-point Likert scale whereas the authors utilized a five-point Likert scale, the mean levels are not comparable. Nonetheless, we still retrieved the general orientation of the schedule by observing positive affect slightly surpassing the expected value with $Mean = 4.75 > 3.50$ and negative affect fractionally undermatching it with $Mean = 3.11 < 3.50$.

With respect to the processual character of the data, we regarded two distinct estimators to assess reliability, that is, internal consistency and split-half reliability. Internal consistency was evaluated by computing Cronbach's α coefficient for each respective variable. Regarding overall art-of-living with $\alpha = .92$, the statistic aligns with preliminary results reported in Chap. 2. Considering art-of-living subscales, the statistics generally ranked at $\alpha \geq .60$ with the exception of "openness" which scored at $\alpha = .52$. Item-total correlations between the subscales and overall art-of-living ranked at the upper range with $r > .50$, indicating a strong relationship between the subscales and the aggregated art-of-living score. Moreover, although the subscales consisted of merely two discriminative items, the respective coefficients align with the statistics reported in Chap. 2. Thus, in addition to the questionnaire, the diary represents a reliable and economical instrument to assess art-of-living. Considering the SWLS, our results ($\alpha = .90$) accord with the statistics reported by the authors ($\alpha = .92$). Also, negative affect ($\alpha = .80$) aligns with the results provided by the authors ($\alpha = .86$) while positive affect ($\alpha = .64$) undermatches the reported statistic ($\alpha = .85$).

To address split-half reliability, we computed stability coefficients following the implications of Schmitz and Skinner (1993). By this means, temporal stability of a given characteristic, that is, estimation of change within the characteristic over the course of a process, can be evaluated. Stability coefficients were estimated for each respective variable by correlating the first half of the process with the second half. Overall, the statistics ranged between $r_{min} = .79$ and $r_{max} = .96$, indicating high stability for all measures covered in the diary. Consequentially, the measures were not generally subject to heavy fluctuations but rather represented consistent trajectories.

Altogether the diary accords with current demands in psychometrics and generally aligns with preliminary work. Thus, we argue that the diary can be utilized as both reliable and economic tool to assess art-of-living and well-being in short-term trajectories.

4.3 Results

Alexander Stahlmann

4.3.1 Validation of the Diary

As a first step, we evaluated the question whether diary and questionnaire yield comparable results. For that purpose, we related individual scores from the diary to the respective scores in the pretest and posttest. To match the process data with the questionnaire, we computed temporally mean level statistics of all measures for the particular participant and the subscale in question each. Subsequently, we correlated the individual mean level statistics with the respective pretest and posttest scores. These results as well as the retest-reliability between pretest and posttest are displayed in Table 4.2.

On the whole, diary and questionnaire exhibited a strong relational framework which reflects in statistically significant relationships within every subscale. Compared to the pretest, the correlation averaged at $r = .61$ while in comparison with

Table 4.2 Correlations of temporally aggregated scores obtained from the diary with the art-of-living questionnaire (pretest and posttest) and retest reliabilities computed as correlation of pretest and posttest scores

Scale	Correlation of diary with pretest	Correlation of diary with posttest	Correlation of pretest with posttest
Coping	.68**	.57**	.76**
Openness	.47**	.42**	.86**
Self-determined way of living	.72**	.68**	.83**
Savoring	.64**	.80**	.83**
Serenity	.56**	.57**	.80**
Balance	.26*	.47**	.49**
Social contact	.45**	.53**	.84**
Self-knowledge	.54**	.72**	.75**
Shaping of living conditions	.54**	.66**	.75**
Physical care	.52**	.63**	.79**
Optimization	.51**	.55**	.65**
Self-efficacy	.67**	.67**	.89**
Positive attitude towards life	.72**	.73**	.88**
Overall art-of-living	.82**	.81**	.90**
SWLS	.76**	.80**	.86**

Explanatory note ** $p < .01$; * $p < .05$

the posttest, it even settled at $r = .66$. Correlation coefficients generally surpassed $r_{min} = .40$ with the exception of "balance", which merely hit $r = .26$ in the comparison between diary and pretest. Especially overall art-of-living achieved high validity coefficients with $r = .82$ in comparison with the pretest and $r = .81$ in comparison with the posttest. In addition, the SWLS also yielded high correlations with $r = .76$ in comparison with the pretest and $r = .80$ in comparison with the posttest.

Based on the comprehensive pretest and posttest protocol, we were also able to address retest reliability within the art-of-living questionnaire and thus further enrich the evidence of psychometric properties reported in Chap. 2. Primarily, correlation coefficients reached $r_{min} = .65$ at least and averaged at $r = .81$. Again, the subscale "balance" represents an outlier as the retest reliability hardly hit $r = .49$. Consequently, the subscale "balance" seems to be subject to certain changes between pretest and posttest. However, as the high split-half reliability coefficients reported earlier in this chapter suggest, the respective temporal trajectory measured by the diary is highly stable. Thus, concerning "balance", although the extent of change between pretest and posttest differs inter-individually, every participant seems to experience similar consistency within the change process. Eventually, overall art-of-living achieved the highest correlation coefficient with $r = .90$ while the SWLS scored at $r = .86$.

Taken together, these findings suggest that diary and questionnaire both yield comparable results. Thus, we can justify the application of the diary as an instrument to assess art-of-living and well-being in short-term trajectories. Furthermore, we showed that art-of-living can be assessed validly by different instruments. On the whole and with the exception of the subscale "balance", art-of-living seems to constitute a stable, temporally more or less consistent trait or attitude rather than an unstable, temporally inconsistent state. Still, individual art-of-living seemed to be subject to a certain amount of change over the course of data acquisition. To evaluate the pattern in change and relate it to preliminary findings, we will subsequently appraise the relationships of art-of-living with current events and well-being.

4.3.2 *Relationship Between Art-of-Living, Current Events and Applied Strategies*

In the framework of positive psychology and health studies, there is great consensus that current events, that is, positive experiences (i.e. uplifts) and negative incidences (i.e. hassles), account for a substantial amount of variation in the daily appraisal of well-being (Diener et al. 1999). In fact, situational factors are reported to even supersede important life events such as marriage, childbirth or the death of a close relative in terms of the relative impact on short-term trajectories in well-being and physical health (DeLongis et al. 1982). However, most of the studies published in recent journals are confined to simple cross-sectional designs and only capture current events in retrospect. To omit these shortcomings, O'Connor et al. (2008) developed short measures of daily uplifts and hassles which were assessed via diary. As the authors showed, particularly daily hassles were related to unhealthy eating behavior. To evaluate the relationship between current events and art-of-living, we assessed both quantity and quality of daily uplifts and daily hassles and correlated the respective scores with overall art-of-living. In addition, we also related the daily amount of applied art-of-living strategies to the overall score. The results are depicted in Table 4.3.

As our findings suggest, overall art-of-living is associated with both quantity (r = .159) and quality (r = .270) of daily uplifts but is not related to daily hassles at all. In addition, overall art-of-living also correlated with the count of applied

Table 4.3 Correlations of overall art-of-living with daily uplifts and hassles as well as the total count of applied art-of-living strategies

	Uplifts (quantity)	Uplifts (quality)	Hassles (quantity)	Hassles (quality)	Art-of-living strategies
Overall art-of-living	.159**	.270**	.001	.002	.255**

Explanatory note ** $p < .01$; * $p < .05$

art-of-living strategies with $r = .255$. Consequently, on a daily base, a high score in overall art-of-living generally co-occurred with a high amount of daily uplifts, a certain importance of the respective events as well as a high amount of applied strategies. However, we cannot assume that art-of-living predicts daily uplifts and applied strategies or vice versa as the correlation statistics do not come up to the requirements of inferences concerning causality. Yet, in principle, causal inferences in process analyses are possible as we will show in the further course of this chapter.

Taken together, we could provide evidence that not only variation in well-being but also in art-of-living is associated with current events. In particular, daily uplifts constituted considerable relationships with art-of-living whereas daily hassles seemed to form no relationship at all. These results only partially accord with the findings reported by preliminary work as most of the studies reported a high negative relationship between well-being and daily hassles but rather low contingencies with daily uplifts (cf. DeLongis et al. 1982; Diener et al. 1999). Yet, although related, art-of-living and well-being constitute two distinct constructs. In the following sections, we will further investigate the precise relational pattern of the two variables. For that purpose, we will firstly evaluate synchronous temporal relationships and subsequently discuss possible antecedents of well-being

4.3.3 Synchronous Relationships Between Art-of-Living, Affect, and Well-Being

In contrast to usual cross-sectional designs, process analyses offer diversified estimators to evaluate the relational framework within a given set of variables over a certain course of time. Generally, two broad categories with divergent objectives are represented by *intra-individual correlations* and *inter-individual correlations*.

To compute intra-individual correlations for a specific participant, the respective trajectories of two variables are correlated temporally. By this means, the within-person relationship of two variables is assessed exclusively for the respective participant. Thus, intra-individual correlations truly capture the individual co-occurrence of two variables within the scope of measurement (i.e. a daily base). In contrast, inter-individual correlations are computed by temporally averaging the trajectories of two variables for each participant and proximately correlating these aggregates. Hence, the between-person relationship of two variables is assessed. Therefore, inter-individual correlations capture the co-occurrence of two variables within a specific sample of participants.

Based on our own data from the diary, we computed both intra-individual as well as inter-individual correlations between art-of-living, well-being and positive and negative affect. To compare both estimators on the level of the whole sample, we computed the mean intra-individual correlation by taking the average of the Fisher's Z-transformed original coefficients. Thus, we assessed the mean

Table 4.4 Three comparable estimators for temporal relationships between art-of-living, well-being and affect

	Mean intra-individual correlation	Mean inter-individual correlation	Intra-individual chain correlation
SWLS	.80**	.84**	.84**
PANAS—positive affect	.68**	.75**	.75**
PANAS—negative affect	−.58**	−.72**	−.72**

Explanatory note ** $p < .01$

relationship between art-of-living and well-being in the trajectories of the sample. In addition, we calculated the intra-individual chain correlation by relating all 1484 observations together. The respective coefficient represents an additional estimator to approach the mean co-occurrence of two variables within a sample over time by treating every observation of each participant and for each occasion as a distinct case (cf. Schmitz and Wiese 2006). The results are depicted in Table 4.4.

In all estimations, art-of-living exhibited high positive synchronous relationships with both the SWLS as well as the positive affect schedule while displaying high negative relationships with the negative affect schedule. These findings generally align with the high correlations between art-of-living and well-being reported in Chap. 3. However, mean inter-individual correlations as well as intra-individual chain-correlations scored substantially higher than the mean intra-individual correlations. These outcomes suggest that the temporal mean levels in art-of-living and well-being are largely comparable across the sample. Yet, intra-individual correlations seem to vary essentially between the participants. Specifically, with respect to the SWLS, intra-individual correlations ranged between $r_{min} = .38$ and $r_{max} = .93$. Hence, although all participants exhibited a certain relational pattern between the two variables, within the trajectories of some particular participants, the relationship was weaker than expected. These findings are illustrated in Fig. 4.1 which depicts the trajectories of art-of-living and well-being for two persons incorporating the lowest and the highest intra-individual correlation coefficients throughout the sample.

On the whole, based on the data obtained from the diaries, we could replicate the high correlations reported in the validation studies. However, methods only executable within the framework of process analyses exposed substantial individual differences in the relationship between art-of-living and well-being. These findings suggest that not generally a high level in art-of-living co-occurs with a high level of well-being but rather that the relationship is shaped by individual characteristics. To approach these attributes, we will evaluate individual mechanisms of causation as a predictor of divergence in the subsequent section.

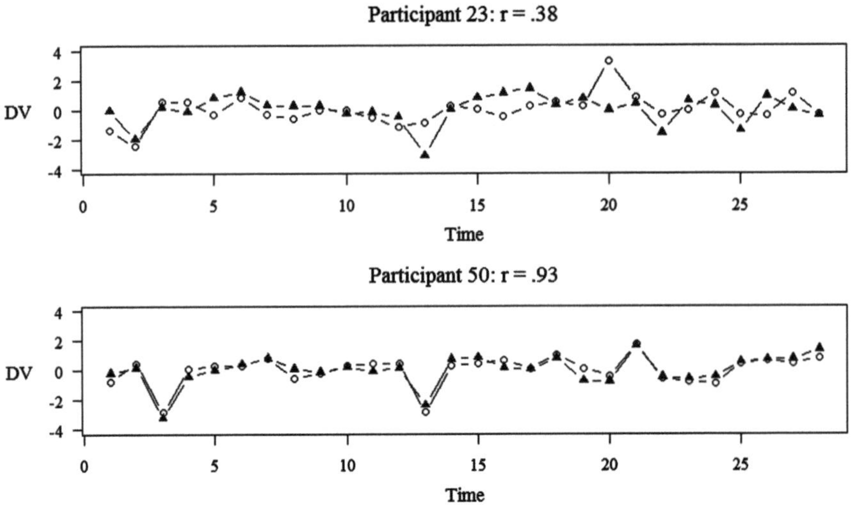

Fig. 4.1 Synchronous relationships between art-of-living (*triangles*) and well-being (*circles*) for participants 23 and 50. Both scales were standardized

4.3.4 *Asynchronous Relationships Between Art-of-Living and Well-Being*

To explain human disparity, that is, to identify and describe the causation for differences in affect, cognition, and behavior is one of the main objectives of psychological research. As noted by Cook et al. (1979), simple correlations do not satisfy this claim as they only capture the strength of synchronous dependence between presumed cause and effect. Furthermore, they call for temporal precedence of the cause, as well as the certainty to exclude alternative explanations for the effect. However, as Granger (1980) notes, this nominal definition lacks applicability and cannot be adopted easily by applied research. Hence, he suggests a functional definition, stating a variable X as causal to a second variable Y if X can explain a significant amount of variance in Y (i.e. Y is regressed by X). In the framework of psychological process analysis Schmitz (1989) approaches the granger-causality by the concept of time-lagged incremental forecasting. By this means, a variable X is forecasted by a second variable Y if there is a strong unidirectional relationship between Y at time t and X at time $t - k$ while k denotes the respective backshift in time t (i.e. temporal precedent variation in X influences current variation in Y). As long as alternative explanations for the relationship are ruled out, time-lagged incremental forecasting provides strong evidence for causality, representing one of the most powerful methods in process analysis.

In exploring the pattern of cause and effect between art-of-living and well-being we analyzed time-lagged incremental forecasting in our diary data. For this purpose, we used vector autoregressive models (VAR-models) implemented by Pfaff (2008)

to compute time-lagged relationships while simultaneously controlling for within-person inertia and synchronous relationships. However, with respect to individual trajectories, $n = 50$ participants (94.34 %) did not show any significant asynchronous relationships between art-of-living and well-being. Considering the remaining participants, all asynchronous regressions were obscured by individual auto-regressions and thus providing no apparent hints regarding causation.

Overall, our results do support the hypothesis that art-of-living and well-being are strongly correlated. Yet, we also reported substantial individual differences in the relationship between art-of-living and well-being. We will subsequently focus on an additional predictor of individual disparity, that is, dynamics in short-term trajectories.

4.3.5 Relationship Between Dynamics in Affect and Overall Well-Being

Whereas cross-sectional psychological research is often confined to point estimations of human characteristics, process analyses offer description, explanation and even forecast of individual development patterns. In process analyses, long-term change is usually approached by tracing shifts in the temporal mean level via regression analyses or by simply computing the mean level statistics. However, to model an appropriate prediction of individual development, one must also take into account the temporal fluctuations framing the mean change of processes.

In a recent issue, Houben et al. (2015) emphasized the relevance of these fluctuations and augmented the common approach with a depiction of three indicators of process dynamics. These indicators are discussed as distinct characteristics of individuals and comprise *process variability*, *process instability* and *process inertia*.

Process variability is introduced as the range on which a process changes over time and usually computed via temporal standard deviation. Therefore, participants exhibiting a high process variability more often reach extreme scores in dependence of their individual mean level. Furthermore, process instability is described as the degree of change from a given moment to the subsequent occasion and often estimated via MSSD (mean-squared-successive-score). The statistic is calculated by averaging the squared (or absolute) difference between every two consecutive occasions. Consequently, participants showing a high process instability undergo major shifts between every successive occasion and thus shape a more unstable process. Process inertia is referred to as the extent to which the level of the previous occasion influences the current development and is usually computed via autocorrelation. By this means, process inertia also describes the degree of alternation of positive and negative shifts between every two successive occasions. Thus, participants incarnating high process inertia can show a lower frequency of variations in positive and negative shifts.

As the authors have shown, all three indicators of process dynamics, computed for negative and positive affect, correlated negatively with temporally aggregated

Table 4.5 Correlations of process dynamics and well-being

	Mean: WB	Pretest: WB	Posttest: WB
Variability: LK	.16	.05	.17
Variability: PA	.00	−.05	.03
Variability: NA	.11	.01	.06
Instability: LK	.09	−.06	.01
Instability: PA	−.14	−.14	−.11
Instability: NA	−.04	−.14	−.07
Inertia: LK	.07	.19	.32 *
Inertia: PA	.25‘	.15	.20
Inertia: NA	.24‘	.12	.16

Explanatory note ‘ $p < .10$; * $p < .05$

well-being. Hence, in terms of forecasting, they argued that a low degree of process dynamics generally predicted a high level of well-being (Houben et al. 2015).

Based on our own data from the diary as well as the pretest and posttest protocol, we also investigated the relationship between process dynamics and overall well-being. In doing so, we computed the three indicators of process dynamics for positive and negative affect as well as for art-of-living. We correlated these indicators with the temporal mean levels of well-being just as with the well-being score extracted from the pretest and posttest protocol. The results are shown in Table 4.5.

Overall, just the correlation between process inertia with respect to art-of-living and well-being in the posttest achieved statistical significance with $r = .32$ and $p < .01$. Besides two more marginally significant contingencies between process inertia of positive and negative affect, no further correlation yielded significant effects. Considering process variability, our results do not align with the findings of Houben et al. (2015), who noted a negative effect with $\hat{p} = -.178$ while, concerning positive and negative affect, our data suggests no relationship. With regards to process instability, our data yields an average correlation of $r = -.14$ for positive affect and $r = -.13$ for negative affect which describe a small effect, but are in accordance with the preliminary finding of $\hat{p} = -.205$. Eventually considering process inertia, we observed a diametrically opposed effect with an average correlation of $r = .20$ for positive affect and $r = .17$ for negative affect while Houben et al. (2015) noted a negative effect with $\hat{p} = -.151$. Altogether, we could only partially confirm the preliminary work; specifically process inertia did not align with our expectations.

These results correspond to the findings depicted in inter-correlation Table 4.6. Whereas all measures of process variability and process instability show medium to large inter-correlation effect sizes, contingencies between process inertia in art-of-living as well as positive affect and the other two indicators generally yielded no effects or even negative correlations. Only process inertia in negative affect formed an exception and exhibited overall a positive relationship with process variability and process instability while simultaneously maintaining a positive correlation with process inertia in positive affect.

Table 4.6 Inter-correlations of process dynamics

	1	2	3	4	5	6	7	8	9
Variability: LK	1								
Variability: PA	.50*	1							
Variability: NA	.62*	.64 *	1						
Instability: LK	.89*	.41 *	.55 *	1					
Instability: PA	.44*	.77 *	.59*	.41*	1				
Instability: NA	.44*	.47 *	.81*	.43*	.66*	1			
Inertia: LK	−.11	.09	−.15	−.42*	−.02	−.12	1		
Inertia: PA	−.03	.20	−.08	−.07	−.33*	−.34*	.32*	1	
Inertia: NA	.30*	.46 *	.31 *	.26 ‘	.23 ‘	−.13	−.04	.34*	1

Explanatory note ‘ $p < .10$; * $p < .05$

Our findings lead to the conclusion that, in contrast to the argumentation of Houben et al. (2015), the foremost three indicators of process dynamics might actually only incorporate two distinct factors, as process variability and process instability share a great amount of common variation. Thereby, these two factors only encompass process inertia as estimation for the density of alternations of positive and negative shifts as well as process variability as an approximation of the range in which these shifts occur. By this means, we can describe process inertia and process variability in accordance with the terms of frequency and amplitude in classical physics, constituting the two main characteristics of process dynamics. Figure 4.2 illustrates four simulated processes and their respective trajectories. One can see that, given the characteristics of the simulation, the two indicators are largely independent: modifying the autocorrelation coefficient does not greatly alter the variance while a variation in variance does not majorly affect the autocorrelation

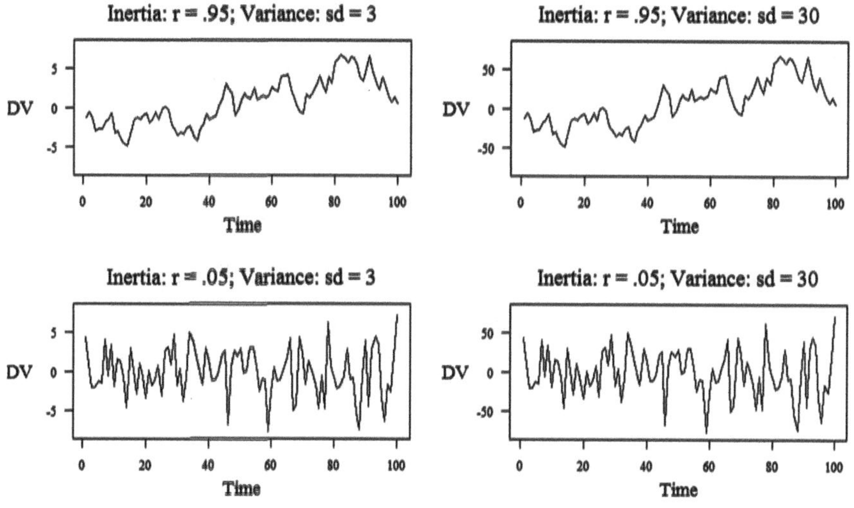

Fig. 4.2 Simulated trajectories in dependence of inertia and variability

coefficient. In contrast, an alteration of variance entails a corresponding shift in the MSSD score. Although the simulation does not come up to the requirements of a formal mathematical proof as it lacks generalizability, the depiction aligns with our results and seems to illustrate the prevailing independence of both estimators.

Altogether, our results depict a composite image. The findings of Houben et al. (2015) could be replicated partially. Although not in complete accordance with preliminary research, these findings consolidate the qualification of process dynamics as justifiable predictor well-being.

4.4 Summary and Overall Discussion

Alexander Stahlmann

In this chapter, we augmented established cross-sectional designs with process analyses to assess trajectories in art-of-living and identify possible antecedents of well-being. For that purpose, we evaluated processual data provided by an extensive diary study and related the results to the respective scores in the art-of-living questionnaire.

Considering psychometric properties, we showed that the diary both economically and reliably captures overall level and short-term trajectories in art-of-living and well-being. Furthermore, the high stability and validity coefficients suggest that mean values across time for art-of-living constitute a stable, temporally consistent trait or attitude. The variation across time (state) shows also systematic covariation over time. In accordance with preliminary research, current important events comprised strong relationships with art-of-living. To investigate the relationship between these trajectories in art-of-living and well-being, we evaluated both intra-individual as well as inter-individual synchronous correlations. As expected the correlation coefficients generally hit high scores, but the intra-individual correlation coefficients differed substantially across the sample. To explain the disparity, we computed asynchronous causation models and examined process dynamics, focusing on the respective individual trajectories. While the asynchronous analyses yielded no compelling results, process dynamics, especially process inertia correlated with well-being constitute a promising approach to describe inter-individual differences in the relational pattern between art-of-living and well-being.

Overall, our results show that process analyses depict an advantageous complement to cross-sectional designs. In particular, process analyses offer a precise evaluation of individual trajectories which are otherwise beyond the scope of measurement. Furthermore, asynchronous models regarding causation and process dynamics can be assessed. Nevertheless, the present study does not ultimately address every research question. Although process inertia seems to predict well-being, the precise causal mechanism is still subject to prospective research. In particular, it is yet unclear whether the three indicators constitute strong or rather weak inter-correlations as our results did not align with the findings reported by Houben et al. (2015). Moreover, our findings raise the question whether process dynamics are confined on specific variables or rather represent a general individual attribute, that is, a latent meta-trait which condenses in several unique characteristics. However, to address and eventually solve these questions, we consider diary studies as a both comprehensive and promising approach for future research.

With respect to the validation of our art-of-living questionnaire, by the diary instrument we added a different method to measure art-of-living. Considering the coefficients in Table 4.2 we found convincing results that the questionnaire and the dairy lead to similar results. Thus, in addition to the peer-ratings of art-of-living and the situational judgement test (SJT) reported in Chap. 3, we presented another valid method to assess art-of-living.

Acknowledgments We would like to thank Boyan Ventsislavov Dimov for the development of the diary and the conduction of the initial study.

References

Cook, T. D., Campbell, D. T., & Day, A. (1979). *Quasi-experimentation: Design & analysis issues for field settings* (Vol. 351). Boston: Houghton Mifflin.

DeLongis, A., Coyne, J. C., Dakof, G., Folkman, S., & Lazarus, R. S. (1982). Relationship of daily hassles, uplifts, and major life events to health status. *Health Psychology, 1*(2), 119–136.

Diener, E. D., Emmons, R. A., Larsen, R. J., & Griffin, S. (1985). The satisfaction with life scale. *Journal of Personality Assessment, 49*(1), 71–75.

Diener, E. D., Suh, E. M., Lucas, R. E., & Smith, H. L. (1999). Subjective well-being: Three decades of progress. *Psychological Bulletin, 125*(2), 276–302.

Glaesmer, H., Grande, G., Braehler, E., & Roth, M. (2011). The German version of the satisfaction with life scale (SWLS). *European Journal of Psychological Assessment, 27*(2), 127–132.

Granger, C. W. (1980). Testing for causality: A personal viewpoint. *Journal of Economic Dynamics and control, 2*, 329–352.

Honaker, J., King, G., & Blackwell, M. (2011). Amelia II: A program for missing data. *Journal of Statistical Software, 45*(7), 1–47.

Houben, M., Van Den Noortgate, W., & Kuppens, P. (2015). The relation between short-term emotion dynamics and psychological well-being: A meta-analysis. *Psychological bulletin, 141* (4), 901–930.

Krohne, H. W., Egloff, B., Kohlmann, C. W., & Tausch, A. (1996). Untersuchungen mit einer deutschen Version der "Positive and negative affect schedule" (PANAS). *Diagnostica, 42*(2), 139–156.

O'Connor, D. B., Jones, F., Conner, M., McMillan, B., & Ferguson, E. (2008). Effects of daily hassles and eating style on eating behavior. *Health Psychology, 27*(1Suppl.), S20–31.

Pfaff, B. (2008). VAR, SVAR and SVEC models: Implementation within R package vars. *Journal of Statistical Software, 27*(4), 1–32.

Schmitz, B. (1989). *Einführung in die Zeitreihenanalyse: Modelle, Softwarebeschreibung, Anwendungen*, Bern: Huber.

Schmitz, B., & Skinner, E. (1993). Perceived control, effort, and academic performance: Interindividual, intraindividual, and multivariate time-series analyses. *Journal of Personality and Social Psychology, 64*(6), 1010.

Schmitz, B., & Wiese, B. S. (2006). New perspectives for the evaluation of training sessions in self-regulated learning: Time-series analyses of diary data. *Contemporary Educational Psychology, 31*(1), 64–96.

Watson, D., Clark, L. A., & Tellegen, A. (1988). Development and validation of brief measures of positive and negative affect: the PANAS scales. *Journal of Personality and Social Psychology, 54*(6), 1063–1070.

Chapter 5
Interventions to Enhance Art-of-Living

5.1 Comparison of a Cognitive and a Combined Cognitive/Body-Related Intervention for Enhancing Art-of-Living and Happiness

Julia Ankenbrand, Bernhard Schmitz

5.1.1 Introduction

"By changing our thinking, we change our lives."

Buddha

According to Sonja Lyubomirsky (2008), to convey a positive attitude towards life and to help people to live a happy life is just as important as the alleviation of mental illness. This approach, both to resolve problems and to improve the well-being, is not new. Already in 1948 the World Health Organization defined health as a "state of complete physical, mental and social well-being and not merely the absence of disease or infirmity" (World Health Organization 1948). The present study is focused on the part of health, which goes beyond the absence of disease or infirmity. That means the focus is on the promotion of the positive aspects of life.

Between 1981 and 2007, the subjective well-being increased in 40 of 52 nations and decreased in the remaining 12 states (Inglehart et al. 2008). Germany was one of the few nations with a decreasing trend (Inglehart et al. 2008). On the "World Map of Happiness" Denmark was ranked 1st and Germany was ranked 35th out of 178 nations (University of Leicester 2006). Therefore the Germans have a great need to become happier, in order to close the gap on their neighboring German-speaking nations.

B. Schmitz, *Art-of-Living*, Social Indicators Research Series 63,
DOI 10.1007/978-3-319-45324-8_5

Art-of-living helps to be happy (Veenhoven 2003a, b). To increase the skills of art-of-living and thus to help people to lead a happy and healthy life, a training for enhancing the art-of-living was developed, implemented and evaluated in the present study.

In the following, art-of-living is defined and the current state of research on art-of-living is presented. Subsequently, *positive attitude towards life* as the focus of the training, is defined and its importance is explained—in particular the benefits of optimism. Furthermore, the influence of intentional actions on the level of happiness is represented as well as interventions of previous studies. Finally, the research question and the hypothesis are formulated.

5.1.1.1 Art-of-Living

"Art-of-living is not understood here as the easy andcarefree life" (Schmid 2007, p. 9), but the conscious, reflective, active and chosen way of life (Schmid 2007) cf. Chap. 1. It is laborious and challenging, but at the same time it leads to a fulfilled and happy life (Schmid 1998, 2007; Veenhoven 2003a; Fellmann 2009). The term "art-of-living" is made up of the words life and art, whereby Schmid (2007) understands *art* as something which is challenging and skillful and *life* as the material of the art (Schmid 1998). Thus being an artist of living is not easy, it is difficult (Schmid 2007). The first step of art-of-living is the decision to walk this path that is open to everyone (Schmid 2007). Everybody can "be the artist and make his life a work of art" (Schmid 1998, p. 75). On the question what you can do for it, Schmid (1998) mentioned the implementation of exercises and the use of techniques. It is about lifelong learning (Schmid 1998). According to Veenhoven (2003b), an intervention to art-of-living is well feasible, because appropriate skills can be learned to some extent. Therefore it is worthwhile, first to know which skills these are and then how they can be improved (Veenhoven 2003b). In previous studies (Chap. 2), the original questionnaire about art-of-living was developed and it consists of 14 components, such as for example *positive attitude towards life*. The development of a training for enhancing these subcomponents, which means the improvement of art-of-living is the main aim of the present study.

5.1.1.2 Positive Psychology

The research on art-of-living belongs to the field of positive psychology. Positive psychology is based on the exploration of positive emotions, positive characters and positive institutions (Seligman and Csikszentmihalyi 2000). The positive emotions include joy, flow, pleasure, satisfaction and serenity (Seligman 2004). After the broaden-and-build-theory of Fredrickson (1998, 2001) positive emotions broaden our mental horizon, which means our thoughts and behavior patterns, and build up our resources, which means our physical, mental and social skills. Positive interventions are aimed at bringing about positive emotions, positive behavior or positive thoughts (Sin and Lyubomirsky 2009). The present study examined whether art-of-living can be enhanced through positive interventions.

5.1.1.3 Positive Attitude Towards Life

Of particular importance to the conception of art-of-living is the subscale *positive attitude towards life*, since it highly correlates with the total value of the art-of-living (r = .80) (Chap. 2). Therefore and because the conveying of a *positive attitude towards life* is important (Lyubomirsky 2008), the focus of the training was directed at *positive attitude towards life*. With respect to a time perspective this means regarding the past, inter alia gratitude, with regard to the present for example joy and in view to the future, for instance optimism (Seligman 2004).

Why is it desirable to be thankful, happy and optimistic? Due to the reinforcement and appreciation of good memories, gratitude increases the satisfaction with life (Seligman 2004). Furthermore, gratitude increases savoring (Seligman 2004). Joy can increase current happiness and optimistic people are confident and have the expectation that even in difficult situations everything will turn out well (Seligman 2004). In the present study it was investigated whether art-of-living can be enhanced by means of a training which includes interventions on *positive attitude towards life*. The majority of these interventions were referred to optimism.

5.1.1.4 Optimism

Why is it worthwhile to be an optimistic person? Previous research showed that optimists live longer than pessimists (Maruta et al. 2000; Danner et al. 2001). Moreover, they have a higher resilience, which means they will be less probable to become depressed, if a blow or other negative events occur, and are thus better protected against mental illness (Fredrickson et al. 2003; Tugade and Fredrickson 2004). Furthermore, they show better performance at school, in sports and at work and have a better immune system and stronger relationships (Lyubomirsky et al. 2005a; Fredrickson 2011; Seligman 2004). Besides, optimists have a high expectation of self-efficacy (Nürnberger 2010), are happier and act more competently (Lyubomirsky 2008; Nürnberger 2010; Bannink 2012). Optimists are amongst other things happy and active, which are also important characteristics of artists of living. Consequently, optimism has many desirable benefits. Interventions to optimism were therefore considered in the present study as a goal-oriented approach for enhancing the art-of-living.

5.1.1.5 Happiness

Lyubomirsky (2008) understands happiness as the experience of joy and satisfaction and the feeling that life is meaningful and worth living. Well-being compared to happiness includes not only emotional but also physical and mental aspects. Every person is to 40 % the architect of his own fortune, 50 % of the happiness level are genetically determined and only 10 % depend on external circumstances (Lyubomirsky et al. 2005b). That means there are 40 % left for increasing the happiness through intentional actions. Seligman (2012) mentioned three ways to happiness: experience of pleasure, flow and meaning. All three aspects are positively correlated with well-being (Schueller and Seligman 2010). The happiest people are those people who strive for all three aspects, above all flow and meaning (Peterson et al. 2005). The interventions in the present study were intentional actions to all three ways to happiness.

5.1.2 Interventions of Previous Studies

A meta-analysis on 49 studies showed that positive interventions increase well-being and reduce depressive symptoms (Sin and Lyubomirsky 2009). In the following, interventions of previous studies, this training was based on, are listed and the derived exercises are mentioned. First of all, interventions which are focused on cognitions are enumerated and after that body-focused interventions are described.

It is advantageous to be grateful, friendly and focused on positive things and to see success as a persistent and a general competence. Emmons and McCullough (2003) found out that grateful people are more optimistic, satisfied and physically healthier. To write letters of gratitude and to be grateful every day for three things makes people happier and less depressed (Seligman et al. 2005). Therefore, on the subject gratitude, the exercises *letter of gratitude* and *daily gratitude* were taken in the present study. Furthermore, the execution of unexpected kindness can lead to a satisfactory mood (Seligman 2012). Based on this, the exercise *unexpected kindness* on the subject joy was carried out in the present study. The direct focus on positive things can make people optimistic (Diegelmann 2007). Besides, imagining a desirable future and writing down one's own role in it is mood-improving (King 2001; Sheldon and Lyubomirsky 2006). On the basis of this the exercises *ABC of positive things*, *good luck beans*, *comics* and *ideal self* on the subject optimism were integrated in the training, because these exercises are directly focused on positive things, and the latter exercise is focused on the wish-future. In addition, on the subject optimism an exercise to *causal attribution* was carried out. According to Seligman (2011) there are three dimensions for explaining success and failure: (1) stability, (2) globality and (3) internality. Optimistic people see failures as temporary and successes as permanently (Seligman 2011). Based on globality, optimists consider failures as individual cases and generalize successes to other areas of life (Seligman 2011). With regard to the third dimension, internality, optimists explain failures caused by too little effort and successes due to a marked ability (Foersterling 1985). The pessimistic style of explanation for failure and success is exactly the opposite of the optimistic style of explanation with the exception that pessimists attribute success to luck in the dimension of internality (Foersterling 1985). According to Seligman (2011) pessimists can learn to be optimistic.

For the training in the present study, two variants were developed. The above mentioned interventions of previous studies were focused on cognitions. The first training variant is limited to cognitive-focused interventions described so far. However, other studies about positive emotions are focused on body-related interventions. So there are already numerous studies that have shown that both purely cognitive-focused and purely body-focused interventions increase positive emotions and decrease depressive symptoms. The present study is aimed at combining both directions of previous interventions, i.e. cognitive- and body-focused interventions, in one training variant, and it wants to test whether this combination is more effective for enhancing the art-of-living than a training with purely cognitive-focused interventions. Therefore the second training variant includes cognitive-focused as well as body-focused exercises. Moreover, many previous studies include only one intervention, although previous research showed that the implementation of many interventions is more effective (Fordyce 1977). There is already a number of impressive interventions of positive psychology, however, the majority of these interventions are designed to only train a single component (Hone et al. 2014). For that reason, it is of interest to develop a training which combines multiple components of positive psychology. Based on the construct of art-of-living, our goal is to determine which components could be combined to predict well-being effectively, we also aim to develop a training program for different samples based on theoretical assumptions and empirical findings. Studies that involve physical exercises were excluded from a meta-analysis conducted by Bolier et al. (2013). With respect to the holistic approach of art-of-living we assume that body-focused tasks could also be of significance for the improvement of well-being. The combination of physical and cognitive components has not yet been adequately studied. For this reason both training variants of the present study comprise many interventions, i.e. exercises.

In the following, studies with body-focused interventions are listed. They show that the focus on the body can positively influence perception and emotions as well as reduce depressive symptoms. The perception of positive things can be trained through *daily mindfulness of the five senses* (Frank 2010). Therefore the *daily mindfulness of the five senses* was carried out as the first body-focused exercise in the second training variant. Another body-focused exercise was about *movement*, because sports can reduce depressive symptoms (Blumenthal et al. 1999). Furthermore, the facial feedback hypothesis means that activities in the face have an influence on the emotions (Strack et al. 1988). Thereby the activation of the laughing muscles leads to positive emotions (Strack et al. 1988). Another body-focused exercise, namely *smile in the mirror every morning*, was aimed at that. A study showed that an upright posture compared to a stooped posture leads to a greater expression of the positive emotion pride in a situation with positive feedback about the performance (Stepper and Strack 1993). Based on this, an exercise about the topic *upright posture* was carried out in the second training variant, which additionally included body-focused exercises.

One aim of this study is to show that art-of-living can be enhanced by our interventions. Different from previous studies we look at combinations of interventions. Bao and Lyubomirsky (2014), p. 380) argue: „…completing multiple activities at once (unlike most experimental settings where a single activity is completed, one at a time) may lead to larger and longer-lasting happiness boosts".

The two trainings we compare are cognitive and a combination of cognitive and body-related exercises.

With respect to the dependent variables we are mostly interested in art-of-living and therefore, we first analyze a variable from art-of-living which should mirror the effect of the training content which is *positive attitude towards life*. Another broader dependent variable is overall art-of-living which summarizes different strategies and attitudes which may help to lead a good life and other components of art-of-living. As in previous studies we also include measures of happiness, e.g. subjective well-being, happiness, and (low) depression. As additional dependent variable which is not included in the art-of-living variables, but which is similar to *positive attitude towards life* we analyze *optimism*.

To test the short time stability we measure each of the dependent variables in a follow-up test 2 weeks later.

5.1.3 Hypotheses

The main aim of this study was the first development, implementation and evaluation of a training for enhancing the art-of-living. This is significant, because art-of-living leads to a fulfilling and healthy life and thus is positive and desirable (Fellmann 2009; Chap. 2). The research question of the present study was: Is art-of-living trainable through the interventions? Based on previous research the following hypotheses were derived:

(1a) Compared to the group without training the training-groups will increase their art-of-living for the variable which mirrors the supposed effect of the interventions (*positive attitude towards life*).

(1b) Because of the interrelatedness of the art-of-living variables there will also be an effect on other variables of the *art-of-living* and the *overall art-of-living*.

(2) The training will also have an effect on *optimism*.

(3) The training will also have an effect on *happiness, satisfaction with life* and *depression*.

(4) The combined cognitive and body-related training group will have an additional effect on *physical self-care*, *overall art-of-living* and *happiness*, *satisfaction with life* and *depression*.

(5) The training effects will be stable for the follow-up measurement.

5.1.4 Method

5.1.4.1 Experimental Design

The present study was based on a two-factorial experimental design with three factor levels and with repeated measurements (3 groups × 3 times). There were three points of measurement (pre-, post-, follow-up test). The independent variable was the group membership respectively the intervention. The dependent variables were the overall art-of-living and all subscales of art-of-living, in addition *optimism*, *satisfaction with life*, *happiness* and *depressive symptoms* and were measured by a questionnaire. Overall, there were three conditions (see Table 5.1). In the first condition (experimental group 1; EG1) the participants were given a cognitive-focused training and in the second condition (experimental group 2; EG 2) a combination of a cognitive- and body-focused training. The participants of the third condition (control group; CG) were the waiting-control group and received an intervention only after the intervention of the experimental groups was completed and the posttest was conducted. The assignment of the participants to the conditions was randomized.

5.1.4.2 Participants

The participants were recruited mainly at a medium city in Germany contacted by the experimenter by means of posters and email. The inclusion criteria were: (1) minimum age of 18 years and (2) no participation in a therapeutic treatment during the study period. The participation was voluntary. As an incentive to participate 30 Amazon vouchers each worth 25 Euro were raffled. Psychology students got credits for participation.

The sample (N = 72) consisted of 51 women (70.8 %) and 21 men (29.2 %) aged 20–74 years (M = 27.35; SD = 9.22). As the highest level of education 45 participants indicate the state “high school” (62.5 %) and 24 participants indicated “university degree” (33.3 %). Two participants had a vocational training (2.8 %) and one participant had another one taken after the sixth year (1.4 %). The most frequent answer to the question on the current occupation was “student” (n = 56; 77.8 %). 12 participants were employees (16.7 %) and in each case one was

Table 5.1 Experimental conditions

Training		
EG 1: cognitive-focused training	EG 2: cognitive- and body-focused training	CG: no training

"trainee" (1.4 %), "not employed: retired" (1.4 %) and "self-employed" (1.4 %). One participant chose "other" (1.4 %) while applying for an university place. Relating to marital status most participants were in a relationship (n = 41; 56.9 %). 20 participants were single (27.8 %), nine participants were married (12.5 %) and two participants were divorced (2.8 %). Relating to sporting activity 56 participants stated, that they regularly do sports which means at least once a week (77.8 %). The sample sizes of the experimental groups and the control group were $N = 23$ (EG1; 78.3 % women), $N = 24$ (EG2; 75 % women) and $N = 25$ (CG; 60 % women). Three participants took only part in the pretest and were therefore excluded from all data and calculations.

5.1.4.3 Measures

The participants of the experimental group completed the questionnaires in paper form, whereas the participants of the control group filled out the questionnaire online. Previous research showed that both forms, paper/pencil and online, can be used in one study (Brock et al. 2012; Cole et al. 2006). In addition to *art-of-living*, *optimism*, *satisfaction with life*, *happiness* and *depressive symptoms* as well as demographic data and data on sporting activities were collected. In the posttest a manipulation check was additionally executed. It was asked whether and how often the particular exercises were implemented between the two training sessions. In the following, the applied questionnaires are described.

Art-of-Living Questionnaire

The questionnaire measuring the art-of-living questionnaire was used, which is described in Chap. 2 as original form. The total value of art-of-living consists of the total scores of all subscales and showed in the present study a Cronbach‘s α of .96 (posttest). The internal consistencies of the subscales in the pre- and posttest are shown in Table 5.2. Most subscales show satisfactory internal consistency.

All subscales except *social contact* were included in the calculations. The subscale *social contact* was excluded because in both pre- ($\alpha = .53$) and post-test ($\alpha = .52$) the internal consistency was not satisfactory. The subscale *optimization* ($\alpha = .54$; pretest) and *integrating different areas of living* ($\alpha = .51$; posttest) are to be interpreted with caution in the calculations.

Table 5.2 Domains of care, subscales of art-of-living, Cronbach's α of the subscales in the pre- and post-test

Domains of care Subscales of art-of-living	Cronbach's α	
	Pretest	Posttest
Self-care		
Self-determined way of living	.72	.85
Self-efficacy	.87	.91
Self-knowledge	.72	.76
Care of the body		
Physical care	.79	.75
Savoring	.62	.71
Care of the Soul		
Balance	.62	.66
Integration different areas of living	.66	.51
Coping	.71	.75
Care of the mind		
Positive attitude towards life	.81	.87
Serenity	.74	.83
Openness	.69	.70
Optimization	.54	.69
Shaping of living conditions		
Social contact	.53	.52
Shaping of living conditions	.80	.91
Overall art-of-living	.94	.96

Optimism from the Revision of the Life Orientation Test (LOT-R)

The revised Life Orientation Test (Scheier et al. 1994; in the German version of Glaesmer et al. 2008) measures *optimism* and *pessimism*. Due to the focus of the present intervention on *positive attitude towards life* this questionnaire was included in the questionnaire. In each case three items measure the optimism and pessimism value. Four items are fillers and were not evaluated. The items are to be answered on a 5- point answer scale (from 1 = *strongly disagree* to 5 = *strongly agree*). An example for an item is: "I'm always optimistic about my future." Glaesmer et al. (2008) reported acceptable psychometric properties. In the present study, only the optimistic value was included in the calculations, Cronbach's $\alpha = .89$ (posttest).

Satisfaction with Life Scale (SWLS)

The satisfaction with life scale (Diener et al. 1985; in the German version of Glaesmer et al. 2011) was used. It was included because previous research found out a high correlation between art-of-living and *satisfaction with life* ($r = .69$) (Chap. 2). The Cronbach's α in the present study amounts to $\alpha = .86$ (posttest).

Subjective Happiness Scale (SHS)

The Subjective Happiness Scale (Lyubomirsky and Lepper 1999; in the German version of Lyubomirsky 2008) measures by four items the current level of happiness cf. Chap. 3. Because art-of-living should help to be happy (Fellmann 2009), this questionnaire has been integrated. Research results show good psychometric properties (Lyubomirsky and Lepper 1999). The Cronbach's α in the present study was .82 (posttest).

Beck Depression Inventory II (BDI-II)

The revised version of the Beck Depression Inventory (Beck et al. 1996; in the German version of Hautzinger et al. 2009) consists of 21 items that measure the severity of depressive symptoms. Previous research showed a reduction of depressive symptoms in positive interventions (Gander et al. 2012), therefore this questionnaire has been included. The items are represented by a 4-point answer scale with statements that are characterized by ascending severity of the symptoms. An example for an item is: "Sadness: I do not feel sad./I feel sad or unhappy./I am unhappy or sad all of the time and I can't snap out of it./I am so unhappy or sad that I can't stand it." The psychometric properties are very satisfactory (Hautzinger et al. 2009). In the present study the Cronbach's α was .89 (posttest).

5.1.4.4 Procedure

All training sessions were held in small groups with maximum eleven participants at the Psychological Institute of the University. The training consisted of two sessions of 2 h each, including test time. There was a week's interval between the training sessions. During this week participants should perform exercises at home. These exercises were presented and prepared in the first training session. In the second training session further exercises were completely carried out in the session. For each exercise participants were given an exercise sheet with a detailed written instruction. Figure 5.1 gives an overview of the training exercises of the two training variants. Two weeks after the posttest a follow-up test was implemented with both experimental groups for testing follow-up effects. In these 2 weeks it was left to the participants, whether, which and how many times they wanted to carry out the exercises of their training.

The control group completed two online questionnaires (pre- and post-test) during the training phase of the experimental group and then received a 2-h training session, consisting of selected exercises of the training sessions of the experimental groups. The training conception and implementation was based on Perels et al. (2008). The methods and media of the training varied, as this positively affects activation, motivation, attention and participation of the participants (Perels et al.

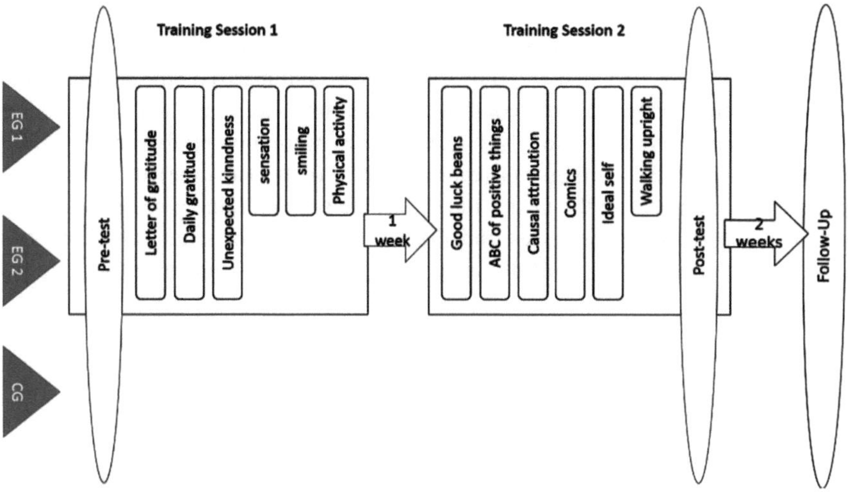

Fig. 5.1 Exercises of both training alternatives

2008). The trainer was supported by an assistant who handed out the materials during the sessions.

Training Session 1, Experimental Group 1: Cognitive Training

The first training session began with the completion of the questionnaire (pretest). This was followed by a warming-up and acquaintance game and questions about the expectations of the training. Then the participants were given an overview of the training, the learning aims were presented and the theoretical knowledge of the art-of-living, *positive attitude towards life*, benefits of optimism and the origin of happiness were conveyed. Following this, exercises were presented and prepared. The first two exercises were about gratitude. The aim of the exercises *letter of gratitude* and *daily gratitude* (cf. Seligman 2004) were the appreciation of good experiences and the reinforcement of positive memories to gain greater satisfaction with the past. The third exercise, *unexpected kindness* (cf. Seligman 2012) was focused on the experience of positive emotions in relation to the present.

Session 1, Experimental Group 2: Cognitive and Body-Related Training

The following exercises of the first training session were body-focused and took place only in the training variant of the experimental group 2. The first body-focused exercise was about *movement* (cf. Blumenthal et al. 1999). The aim of this exercise was to experience flow in the here and now. The exercise *daily mindfulness of the five senses* (cf. Frank 2010) was about the attentive perception of the present. As a final exercise of the first training session *smile in the mirror every morning* (cf. Strack et al. 1988) was represented, with the aim to start the day optimistic. Finally, the first training session was summarized, the learning aims were taken up, a view of the second training session was given and in a flashlight the participants were asked to which exercise they were looking forward most. In a weekly schedule the participants recorded when (date and time) they wanted to perform the exercises in the next 7 days until the second training session. Through the preparation of the exercises and the written record of when which exercise should be carried out in the following week, the transfer into everyday life was ensured.

Session 2, Experimental Group 1: Cognitive Training

The second training session was initiated with the exercise *good luck beans* (cf. Seligman 2004), which accompanied the participants throughout the whole second session. This was followed by a repetition of the first training session as well as a reflection on the exercises, which were presented und prepared in the first session and implemented at home until the second training session. Then the participants were given an overview of the session and the learning aims were presented. This was followed by the *ABC of positive things* (cf. Diegelmann 2007), which had the aim to focus on positive things. As an entry for the second exercise, *causal attribution* (cf. Seligman 2011; Foersterling 1985), the teaching of theoretical knowledge about causal attribution followed. The aim of this exercise was the creation of a consciousness of pessimistic and optimistic causal attribution as well as the ability to convert pessimistic into optimistic statements for explaining success and failure. After showing funny *comics*, the exercise *ideal self* (cf. King 2001) was carried out, in which the participants focused on positive emotions and insights about themselves in relation to the future.

Session 2, Experimental Group 2: Cognitive and Body-Related Training

Then for the training variant of the experimental group 2 the exercise *upright posture* (cf. Stepper and Strack 1993) followed, in which the participants perceived the influence of their body on their emotions. After a summary of the training, which was oriented towards the three paths to happiness (pleasure, engagement and meaning) by Seligman (2012), the learning aims were taken up and the participants were asked in a flashlight which exercise they liked best.

In addition they were asked whether a bean was moved in the exercise *good luck bean* that means whether the participants experienced one or more happy moments during the second training session. Finally, the participants completed the questionnaire (posttest) which had already been used in the pretest. This questionnaire also contained manipulation check questions to assess whether the exercises were actually carried out. Only data from participants who reported to have carried out at least two of the three or four of the six exercises, depending on the training variant, were included in further calculations. No participant had to be excluded from further calculations according to this condition. The follow-up was performed 2 weeks after the post-test.

5.1.4.5 Analyses

First of all, it was tested whether there were differences between the groups in the pretest with respect to the dependent variable by using analysis of variance (Tabachnick and Fidell 2013). In the next steps the data from pre- and post-test were examined. It was tested whether there was a significant interaction time × group by using planned comparisons, one between the combined experimental groups and the control group and the other one between experimental group 1 and 2. Finally the follow-up effects were examined by testing the time (post-test vs. follow-up) × group interaction.

5.1.5 Results

5.1.5.1 Descriptive Results

The mean values and standard deviations of all scales for all groups and the first two measurement time points (pre- and posttest) are listed in Table 5.3. The table shows that the mean values of all scales, with the exception of the scale *depression*, have increased over the time in the two experimental groups. The mean values of the subscale *serenity* have increased only in the group with cognitive- and body-focused training. In addition, the range of values for depressive symptoms shows that there is no depression (Hautzinger et al. 2009). The maximum value in the experimental group 1 was six, in the experimental group 2 five and in the control group seven.

Comparison of the Groups in the Pretest

By using analysis of variance, it was tested with the factor group membership and the scales as dependent variables whether there were significant differences between the groups before training. These calculations showed no significant results. There were thus no significant differences between the groups with respect to the scales in the pretest.

Table 5.3 Means and standard deviations of the three groups and pre- and post-test for all scales

Scales	Experimental group 1				Experimental group 2				Control group			
	Pretest		Posttest		Pretest		Posttest		Pretest		Posttest	
	M	*SD*	*M*	*SD*	*M*	*SD*	*M*	*SD*	*M*	*SD*	*M*	*SD*
Overall art-of-living	4.45	0.54	4.67	0.55	4.39	0.36	4.64	0.41	4.47	0.34	4.47	0.37
Balance	4.53	0.63	4.76	0.67	4.70	0.45	4.97	0.31	4.66	0.65	4.58	0.64
Coping	3.81	0.75	4.10	0.76	3.86	0.67	4.21	0.53	4.01	0.50	4.11	0.60
Serenity	3.64	1.09	3.61	1.29	3.32	0.79	3.72	0.87	3.82	0.81	3.81	0.83
Savoring	4.47	0.74	4.53	0.69	4.29	0.53	4.48	0.54	4.39	0.59	4.30	0.72
Shaping of living conditions	4.92	0.58	5.18	0.68	4.82	0.77	4.97	0.77	4.93	0.56	4.79	0.55
Physical care	4.82	0.79	5.12	0.63	4.74	0.73	4.93	0.55	4.64	0.59	4.61	0.57
Integrating different areas of living	3.74	0.86	3.94	0.72	3.81	0.83	4.01	0.75	3.52	0.86	3.68	0.74
Openness	4.88	0.52	4.99	0.58	4.61	0.59	4.72	0.69	4.59	0.77	4.53	0.62
Optimization	4.05	0.42	4.20	0.41	3.95	0.35	4.19	0.33	4.15	0.35	4.11	0.34
Pos. attitude towards life	4.90	0.77	5.00	0.79	4.85	0.69	4.98	0.60	4.86	0.61	4.75	0.63
Self-knowledge	4.57	0.63	4.93	0.61	4.69	0.48	4.96	0.50	4.88	0.48	4.95	0.44
Self-determined way of living	4.81	0.58	5.06	0.59	4.73	0.52	5.04	0.58	4.77	0.50	4.82	0.53
Self-efficacy	4.32	0.70	4.64	0.63	4.27	0.58	4.60	0.65	4.43	0.58	4.48	0.64
Optimism	4.22	0.84	4.54	0.66	3.99	0.85	4.33	0.71	4.09	0.73	4.09	0.83
Satisfaction	5.32	1.09	5.46	1.15	5.36	1.11	5.76	0.99	5.18	1.08	5.46	0.90
Happiness	5.22	1.27	5.48	1.36	5.39	0.99	5.69	1.03	5.45	1.10	5.43	0.95
Depression	1.30	0.39	1.24	0.39	1.23	0.20	1.16	0.20	1.31	0.28	1.26	0.19

Optimism = Life Orientation Test, Satisfaction = Satisfaction with Life Scale, Happiness = Subjective Happiness Scale, Depression = Beck Depression Inventory

Calculation of the Differences Between Pre- and Posttest for the Control Group and the Experimental Groups

We first test the hypotheses whether the pre-post difference in the two experimental groups significantly differ from the control group. The results of the contrast tests are shown in Table 5.4.

Regarding Hypothesis (1a):

For *positive attitude towards life* there is a significant difference between the experimental groups and the control group *positive attitude towards life*: $t(69) = -3.35$, $p = .001$, $\eta^2 = .18$;

Regarding hypothesis 1b):

For *overall art-of-living* as well as for the subscales *balance*, *savoring*, *shaping of living conditions*, *physical care*, *self-determined way of living* and *self-efficacy*, there exist significant contrasts (see Table 5.4). Note that are also non-significant results for *coping*, *serenity*, *integrating different areas of living*.

Table 5.4 Planned contrasts for the differences between groups for the pre- post-test-differences

Scales	Differences between pre- and posttest					
	Experimental groups versus control group			Experimental group 1 versus experimental group 2		
	t	df	η^2	*t*	df	η^2
Overall art-of-living	−4.78**	69	.31	0.75	69	–
Balance	−3.07**	69	.15	0.34	69	–
Coping	−1.95	69	–	0.53	69	–
Serenity	−1.60	69	–	2.97**	69	.14
Savoring	−2.22**	69	.09	1.15	69	–
Shaping of living conditions	−3.81**	69	.22	−1.10	69	–
Physical care	−3.20**	69	.17	−1.11	69	–
Integrating different areas of living	−0.31	69	–	0.03	69	–
Openness	−2.05*	69	.07	0.03	69	–
Optimization	−3.21**	69	.17	1.05	69	–
Positive attitude towards life	−3.35**	69	.18	0.33	69	–
Self-knowledge	−3.19**	69	.16	−0.99	69	–
Self-determined way of living	−3.24**	69	.18	0.82	69	–
Self-efficacy	−3.94**	69	.23	0.24	69	–
Optimism	−3.17**	69	.16	0.23	69	–
Satisfaction	0.08	69	–	1.88*	69	.06
Happiness	−1.99*	69	.07	0.17	69	–
Depression	1.64	69	–	−0.26	69	–

η^2 = partial eta squared; Optimism = Life Orientation Test, Satisfaction = Satisfaction with Life Scale, Happiness = Subjective Happiness Scale, Depression = Beck Depression Inventory
$^* p \leq .05$; $^{**} p \leq .01$

Note also, that there is a significant difference also for *physical care.*

Hypothesis (2)

The contrast analysis also shows a significant effect for the scale *optimism*: $t(69) = -3.17$, $p = .001$, $\eta^2 = .16$.

Hypothesis (3)

The contrasts is significant for *happiness:* $t(69) = -1.99$, $p = .025$, $\eta^2 = .07$; but not for *satisfaction* and *depression.*

Hypothesis (4)

The contrast between the two experimental groups is not significant for *physical self-care* and *overall art-of-living* and there is no additional effect of the combined cognitive and bodily-related group for *happiness* and *depression.* But there is an effect for *satisfaction with life:* $t(69) = 1.88$, $p = .032$, $\eta^2 = .06$.

Hypothesis (5)

The comparison between post-test and follow-up does not yield any significant difference. Therefore, the results were stable.

The significant contrasts for the dependent variables *overall art-of-living*, *optimism* and *positive attitude towards life* are graphically shown in Figs. 5.2, 5.3 and 5.4. In the graphical representation of the difference between pre-and posttests for the groups the means of the scales *overall art-of-living* and *optimism* of both experimental groups rise from pre- to post-test, whereas the means of the control group remain constant (see Figs. 5.2, 5.3). Moreover, according to Fig. 5.4, the means of the scale *positive attitude towards life* rise in the experimental groups compared to the control group in which the line of the means drops.

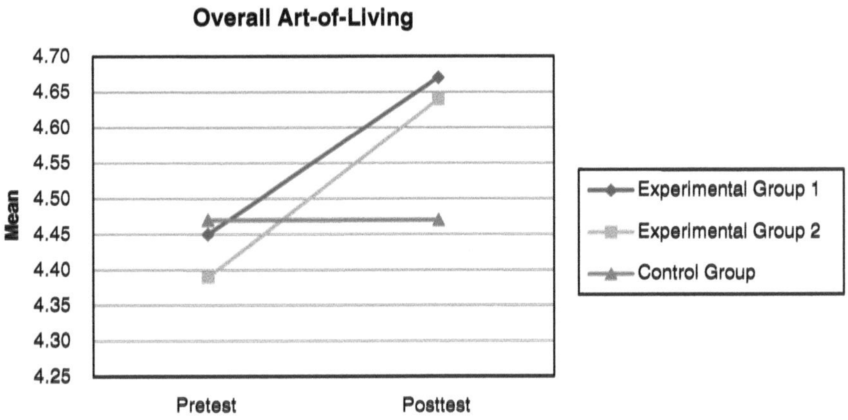

Fig. 5.2 Time × group interaction for *overall art-of-living*

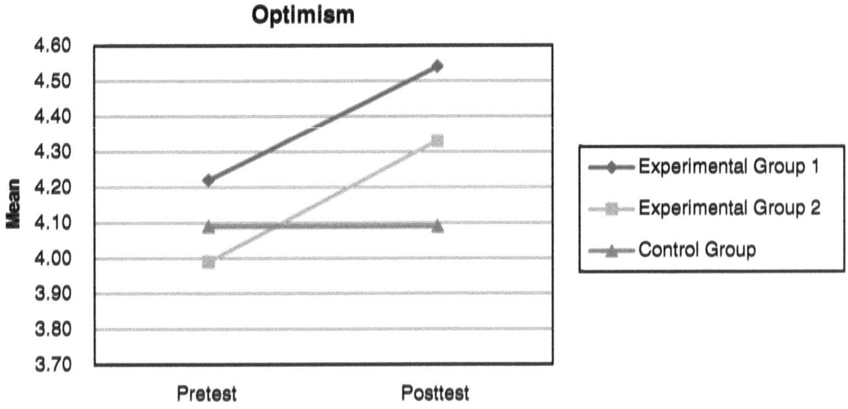

Fig. 5.3 Time × group interaction for *optimism*

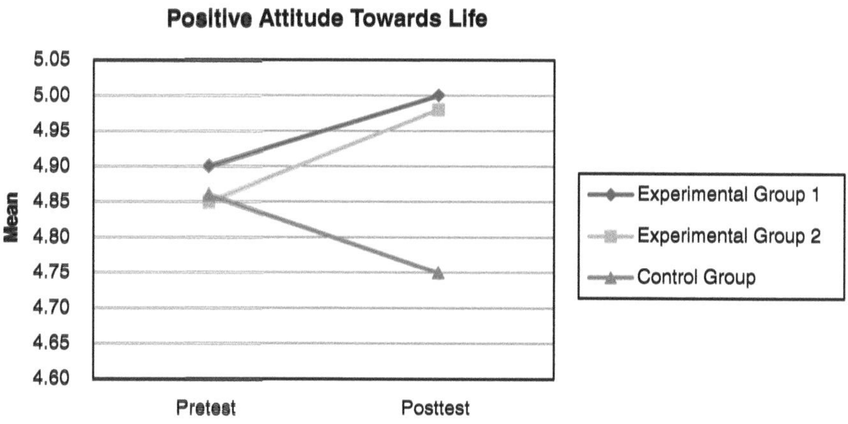

Fig. 5.4 Time × group interaction for *positive attitude towards life*

5.1.6 Discussion

In the present study, a training for enhancing art-of-living was developed, implemented and evaluated. It was especially tested for the first time whether art-of-living can be enhanced by positive interventions. Furthermore, it was investigated in contrast to previous studies whether a training variant that combines cognitive- and body-focused exercises is more effective than a training variant of purely cognitive-focused exercises. In addition, a training with several exercises was developed, since this seems to be more effective (Bao and Lyubomirsky 2014) and more varied and thus the risk of boredom is reduced (Fordyce 1977; Lyubomirsky et al. 2005b). Again whereas previous studies included mostly just one intervention the present study investigates different combinations of exercises. The results indicate that these combinations are highly effective because they allow to enhance not only *positive attitude towards life* but also *overall art-of-living*. That means also, that art-of-living is trainable through interventions that focus on *positive attitude towards life*. In the following, the results related to the hypotheses are discussed and the effect of the training is explained.

First, the results are summarized. The groups with training increased their *positive attitude towards life*. This result was confirmed by another measure *optimism*, which is not contained in the art-of-living questionnaire. Both results combined allow a stable conclusion that our training worked for dependent variables which are related to the training concepts. Of special interest is that the training also enhanced *overall art-of-living* compared to the group without training. Thus art-of-living can be improved by both training variants. Besides, following scales were increased in the groups with training compared to the group without training: *balance*, *savoring*, *shaping of living conditions*, *physical care*, *openness*, *optimization*, *self-determined way of living*, *self-knowledge*, and *self-efficacy*. This is remarkable because although the intervention contains some exercises, its delivery took place only within two short training sessions.

With respect to different measures of happiness the results have to be differentiated. First, happiness measured by the Subjective Happiness Scale (SHS) (Lyubomirsky and Lepper 1999) could be enhanced by the experimental groups. The increase of *happiness* can be explained by the fact that art-of-living is meant to enhance happiness (Fellmann 2009). Moreover, interventions of all three paths to happiness according to Seligman (2012) were carried out.

For subjective well-being (SWLS) (Diener et al. 1985) only the group with cognitive and bodily-related exercises could enhance their well-being. Whereas well-being is an often used measure for positive psychology interventions this result is somewhat unexpected. A detailed look at Table 5.3 shows that this effect might be due to an unexpected high gain in the control group, may be because of instrumentation effects insofar as they might became sensitive for their well-being through the pretest. Also a little bit unexpected is the fact that for depression there is no training effect for both experimental groups. As was already mentioned in the results section, the values for depression for the subjects in all groups are very low. That means the missing reduction in depression could be explained by a floor effect. In sum, it could be concluded that training effects with respect to happiness and satisfaction but not for depression could be observed.

Regarding hypothesis 4 there were only a few differences between cognitive and the combination of cognitive and bodily oriented groups. Both groups were rather effective. That means that the differences between the groups were not very big. The training sessions for both groups were of same length because we did not want to investigate the effect of different time investment but instead the effect of different contents. Both groups received a common package of cognitive exercises and because of the similar effects one might conclude that the common part of the interventions led to the results. Therefore, it might be helpful to add an experimental group with only bodily-related exercises for future studies.

Moreover, the non-significant comparison using the data from post- and follow-up test, revealed that the effect of the training remained stable. Although the distance between posttest and follow-up was short, there are many studies which do not include any follow-up at all. Therefore, our approach was a small step in the right direction.

It can therefore be assumed that a training for *positive attitude towards life* has a positive effect on the art-of-living, many components of art-of-living, *optimism* and *happiness* (cf. Table 5.4). The groups with training could improve their physical (e.g. *physical care*), and mental (e.g. *self-efficacy*) health. Consequently, after the training the groups with training possibly could lead a happier and healthier life than before training.

The effect sizes showed that for the measurement of the dependent variable, the effect of interaction time × group is medium to large. According to Cohen (1988) $\eta^2 = .01$ is a small effect, $\eta^2 = .06$ is a medium effect and $\eta^2 = .14$ is a large effect. The contrast between experimental and control groups explains 31 % of the variance in *overall art-of-living* and 18 % of the variance in *positive attitude towards life* as well as 16 % of the variance in *optimism*. Large effects were also found on the scales *self-determined way of living* and *self-efficacy*. Therefore, the present study exceeds previous studies of positive interventions that showed small to moderate effects (Sin and Lyubomirsky 2009).

An important question is: Why do the interventions that were used in the present study increase the *art-of-living* and the subscales of *art-of-living*, *optimism* and *happiness*? The broaden-and-build-theory of positive emotions of Fredrickson (1998, 2001) serves as a general framework for the interpretation of the results. All used interventions are aimed at inducing positive emotions, which build up physical and mental skills (Fredrickson 1998, 2001). In addition, the increased mindfulness can serve as a further explanation. The focus on positive emotions in the training and exercises can lead to an increased mindfulness of positive emotions in everyday life and therefore the perception of positive emotions is facilitated. Furthermore, the independent implementation of the exercises in everyday life required self-regulatory skills. According to Schmitz and Wiese (2006), reflection plays an important role in self-regulation. A high degree of self-regulation can therefore support a reflected life, which is characteristic for an artist of living, and can help to carry out the effective exercises in everyday life and thereby increase the art-of-living. Thus, self-regulation can also be used to explain the results.

5.1.6.1 Limitations and Future Research Opportunities

In the following, the limitations of this study and future research opportunities are considered. The limitations are the short period of time, no significant reduction of depressive symptoms, no inclusion of a third experimental group, which would receive only body-focused exercises and a control group which would receive an alternative training. In addition, another limitation could be the frequency of the implementation of the exercises and objective assessment methods.

In the present study, a pre-, post- and follow up-test was implemented and thereby a short period of time, which means 4 weeks, was considered. Future studies should examine by means of follow-up investigations whether there are long-term effects after more than 4 weeks. In a study by Seligman et al. (2005) participants also carried out exercises in a week and benefited up to 6 months after the implementation of the exercises, since they voluntarily carried them out after this week. Cohn and Fredrickson (2010) demonstrated long-term effects of positive interventions after 1 year.

The computation of contrasts between experimental and control groups showed no significant effects for the depressive symptoms in the present study. The depressive symptoms could not be reduced by the intervention. This unexpected result can be explained by the fact that the present sample showed no depression. Thus, a positive effect after the examination of the sample was no longer expected. In a study by Gander et al. (2012) and in other studies, the samples showed higher depressive symptoms which could be reduced by intervention (Sin and Lyubomirsky 2009). Moreover, it should be examined whether the training has a preventive effect against depression, which means that training participants are less likely to get depressive. Besides, in future studies the training could be implemented in a clinical sample with increased depressive symptoms in order to investigate whether these could be reduced. Furthermore, the sample consisted of many women and students. Future studies should test the training on a gender-balanced sample as well as on people from different educational levels and ages.

The present study examined the effect of two training variants. The first training variant included cognitive-focused exercises and the second training variant additionally body-focused exercises. Further studies should involve a third training variant, which examines the effect of a pure body-focused training variant, for comparing both the two individual foci as well as the combination of cognitive- and body-focused interventions. Since the group with the cognitive- and body-focused training significantly differed from the group with purely cognitive-focused training only in a few scales, future research should investigate the improvement of the effectiveness of the training variant with cognitive- and body-focused exercises. Moreover, there was only one control group, a waiting control group, in the present study. Another possible control group could get an alternative training for controlling general training effects and Hawthorne effects. In addition, the training variants were implemented in small groups. Future studies should investigate whether different sizes of training groups influence the effects.

Only data from participants who had completed at least two training exercises were included in the calculations. Furthermore, it should be investigated whether the implementation frequency of the exercises has an influence on the effects. The focus of the present intervention is based on *positive attitude towards life*. In future studies it should be tested whether interventions with the focus on other concepts of the art-of-living are also effective or more effective for enhancing art-of-living.

The present study examined the effect of interventions based on self-reports. Further studies should also involve other assessment methods.

5.1.7 Conclusion

The results of the present study lead to the conclusion that it is possible to enhance art-of-living through a training, which is focused on *positive attitude towards life*, by two training sessions and this effect remains stable after a period of 2 weeks.

Different from previous studies we investigated combinations of exercises. The results showed that art-of-living is trainable. It could also been demonstrated that both training variants are very effective for enhancing art-of-living. In addition, *optimism* and *happiness* could also be increased through the training.

5.2 Spoilt for Choice? How Does the Kind of Assignment for Strategies of Art-of-Living Effect Training Results?

Corinna Gräfe

5.2.1 *Introduction*

An impressive number of interventions of positive psychology already exists. But most of them are designed to only train single components and not a combination of multiple components (Hone et al. 2014). Art-of-living is a construct which holistically integrates a large group of variables. It is of interest to develop an intervention which trains not each but a selection of multiple art-of-living strategies. In the past, trainings designed to increase well-being were developed. We also presented a training to enhance art-of-living, cf. Sect. 5.1.Because art-of-living consists of a large group of variables, it is clear that not every strategy can be trained. But how can a selection of strategies be managed? Until now there is no training evaluating the best way of assigning strategies. Therefore, the present study deals with the question, which way of assignment of art-of-living strategies is most effective. Three approaches seem to be theoretically or empirically founded: One assumption is that autonomy with respect to the choice of strategies is most important. This assumption is supported by Ryan and Deci (2000) who found that experiencing autonomy leads to the development of interest and intrinsic motivation for performing the behavior. Following this assumption it would be appropriate to let the subjects choose the strategies. Another option would be that prior research has shown which strategies are most successful and therefore, the kind of strategy is chosen by the researchers based on the results of former studies. A third method of strategy assignment could be that individuals were pretested with respect to their application of strategies. And for the training the kind of strategies are chosen which were until now only rarely applied by the subject. Therefore, in this study it will be tested which of these three kinds of strategy assignments is most effective. To evaluate these kinds of assignment strategies we studied three groups of individuals who attained a different kind of assignment. In addition, a control group did not receive any training. To support the transfer of the training into real life behavior we applied a diary asking for the application of art-of-living strategies. In former studies it was shown that this kind of diary can support the application of strategies into real life contexts (Schmitz and Perels 2011). Regarding the target group we found that there is a discrepancy between empirical research and the idea of establishing interventions of positive psychology in school context. Due to methodical criteria the meta-analysis of Bolier et al. (2013) could not include school-based intervention studies. But the situation faced by students contains an increased pressure to achieve good academic results. Students have also a high prevalence of depression (Seligman et al. 2009). A preventive use of interventions aiming at positive emotions might be necessary (Seligman and Csikszentmihalyi 2000). To learn how to deal with one's self at a young age might be helpful by dealing with life stressors. For that reason, interventions to encourage students in their way of life are of high relevance. Our hypotheses are related to three aspects: the overall effectivity of the training regardless of the strategy assignment, the superiority of the autonomy-based strategy assignment and the enhancement of applying art-of-living strategies during the time-course of the training.

5.2.2 *Hypotheses*

(1) Compared to the control group a significant increase in well-being and the art-of-living-scores can be measured for all types of training.

(2) Based on the theory of Ryan and Deci (2000) and convincingly empirical evidence for their theories it is presumed that the assignment allowing the subject autonomously to select the training strategies will be the most effective training.

(3) Because of the growing effect of the training and supplemented by the transfer support of the diary the daily scores for art-of-living and well-being in the art-of-living-diary show positive trends.

5.2.3 *Method*

The classes were randomly assigned to one of the four experimental conditions (one control and three experimental groups) which were determined by the way of choosing (preselected) strategies (experimental group). All groups participated both in the pre- and in the post-test[1] (see Fig. 5.5).

5.2.3.1 Participants

The sample comprised 164 senior grade students (♀ 58.5 %) from four different schools in Germany. Participants were between 14 and 19 years old. They were offered to participate at a lottery at the end of the study.

[1]It was planned to include a follow-up test but only a small part of the students worked on the follow-up test, therefore we do not present these data.

	Kind of Strategy			
	Pretest	Selection	Training	Postest
Control Group	x	-	-	x
Experimental Group 1	x	Selection 1	X	x
Experimental Group 2	x	Selection 2	X	x
Experimental Group 3	x	Selection 3	X	x

X = Training in art-of-living, Selection 1 = autonomous selection of art-of-living strategies, Selection 2 = Five domains with low art-of-living values, Selection 3 = Three strategies chosen by the experimenter

Fig. 5.5 Design

5.2.3.2 Measures

In order to measure the students' respective art-of-living-score they were asked to answer both the revised questionnaire, s. Chap. 2 and the SWLS, which was used for recording the overall *satisfaction with life.*

Art-of-Living Questionnaire

The used revised questionnaire, is described in Chap. 2. In this study the reliability of the scales lies between .50 and .83. The Cronbach's Alpha of the overall art-of-living is regarded as being high (.87).

Satisfaction with Life Scale (SWLS)

The SWLS is also described in Chap. 2 and shows a Cronbach's Alpha of .75.

Diary

The diary contains 25 questions, among them four concerning well-being, one for each of the 17 art-of-living-scales plus further questions regarding the realization of the strategies. Example question for state well-being "Today, my day was …" ("very good" (6)… "very bad" (1)), example item for art-of-living "Today I know that I self-determine my life" on 6-point Likert-type scales (1 = "strongly disagree"

6 = "I strongly agree"). State art-of-living-total showed satisfactory reliability, $\alpha = .89$ and SWLS state .85.

5.2.3.3 Procedure

The training procedure follows a classical concept derived from Perels et al. (2008) which is adapted from Silberman (1990). Participants are asked to fill out the questionnaire. The three different trainings begin with a short welcoming exercise. Furthermore, the trainer presents information about the art-of-living.

This knowledge enables the identification and analysis of possible art-of-living-strategies. Then, the students assess whether or not they have already implemented various strategies in their everyday lives. Afterwards, participants are introduced to a group of strategies dependent on their experimental group. The application is supported by a diary, which is also available online. The selected art-of-living-strategies benefit from the social context inherent to classes as well as from the daily routine with regard to the academic responsibilities. Nevertheless, strategies that do not directly focus on an academic environment can help to support deficient art-of-living-domains. All participants are supposed to adopt the (chosen) strategies into their everyday lives, individually experiencing the effects. At the end of the training, students are asked to apply their newly acquired knowledge to everyday situations in order to further emphasize their benefit. This also causes the participants to internalize solutions for implementation problems, thereby forwarding the transfer of the strategies into both the private and academic daily routine (Besser 2004).

General Strategies for All Groups

In addition to the instruction how to use the diary for learning and daily life, all students get an introduction in goal-setting and planning. The idea is that goal-setting and planning are strategies that help them to solve problems which are school related but also can be important in private life, e.g. with respect to sports or playing instruments. Goal-setting deals with formulating challenging but realistic and concrete goals. Planning includes to think about time-management and resources necessary for adequately handling their daily tasks, cf. Schmitz and Wiese (2006).

Strategies for Group 1

The students got information about all the strategies which were summarized in Table 5.5. Group 1 could choose autonomously from all strategies.

Table 5.5 Strategies for each component of art-of-living

	Strategy	Source
Coping	Becoming aware of mastered difficult situations; theoretical dealing with strategies	Kaluza (2005) Lyubomirsky (2008)
Openness	Identifying similar daily routines; trying new things; dialectic; talking to new people	Lyubomirsky (2008) Meier (2005)
Self-determined way of living	Realizing desired activities; analyzing the expectations oneself and others have about oneself; changing disruptive situations	Meier (2005)
Savoring	Consciously enjoying agreeable things; remembering agreeable situations; diary with only positive things; taking pictures of beautiful things; writing down agreeable sensory stimuli	Lyubomirsky (2008) Meier (2005) Frank (2010)
Serenity	Short daily timeouts; meditation; yoga; autogenic training; not ruminating about disagreeable things; questioning why one is upset; smiling when waking up	Frank (2010) Seligman (2004) Kaluza (2005) Beitel (1999) Lyubomirsky (2008)
Integrating different areas of life	Comparing actual values to set points of important areas of life; writing a letter to a temporally overrepresented area with reasons why that is no longer possible; imagining a short film about oneself and the perfect day	Frank (2010) Meier (2005)
Balance	Being extreme for 1 week; becoming aware of contrasts between boredom and excessive demands	Schmid (2007) Meier (2005)
Social contact	Well-being ABC; organizing regular meetings; filling in a questionnaire about conflicts; writing letters/postcards; being helpful; taking time for important people	Frank (2010) Beitel (1999) Lyubomirsky (2008)
Self-knowledge	Listing personal preferences; writing an eulogy to oneself; filling in a questionnaire about life energy; reflecting about one's fears	Meier (2005) Frank (2010) Beitel (1999)
Physical care	Body Scanning; making a plan to cook tasty recipes; developing a going-to-bed-ritual; starting to do physical exercise	Frank (2010) Lyubomirsky (2008)
Optimization	Information about time management; Pareto's principle of time; finding time-eaters; ABC-scheme; Eisenhower's principle; keeping a learning diary	Seiwert (1995) Landmann and Schmitz (2007)
Positive attitude towards life	Developing a positive image of the future; promoting gratefulness; thanking others; making ingratitude positive; passing in review positive things before going to bed; paying attention to positive things; writing down especially positive things; having a positive attitude towards one's weaknesses; collecting something	Frank (2010) Lyubomirsky (2008) Seligman (2004) Meier (2005)

(continued)

Table 5.5 (continued)

	Strategy	Source
Shaping of living conditions	Decorating one's flat; tidying up; noticing positive aspects in one's environment	Roth (2007) Beitel (1999)
Self-efficacy	Reaching goals through thoughts; setting a small goal for the near future; thinking of reasons for reaching goals	Pfennig (2009) Schwarzer and Jerusalem (2002)
Self-actualization	Writing down wishes, convictions, needs and how one is acting according to them; goal-directed planning of the week; making a list with strengths and how one can use them	Lyubomirsky (2008) Seiwert (1995)
Reflection	Reflecting which goals one had, whether they were realized and why; Reflecting how one reacts in situations and why; reflecting about things past	Reil (2012)

Strategies for Group 2

The students got information about all the strategies which were summarized in Table 5.5, that are the same strategies as in group 1. As all groups also group 2 has made the pretest for art-of-living. The students from group 2 should choose the strategies for which they have the lowest subtest values.

Strategies for Group 3

In order to give a brief impression over the strategies the students utilized, the five strategies used in training type III are explained below. The strategies were selected from the research team with respect to the estimated utility for school and private life.

Coping.

In the definition of art-of-living *coping* is defined as to deal well with difficult situations. In order to train this component, participants are instructed and guided to become aware of and acknowledge the presence of different alternatives of solving a problem. They are asked to reimagine a difficult or stressful situation they already mastered before contemplating exactly how this situation was resolved and imagining further alternative solutions to a similar problem. Thinking about the considerations leads to a feeling of having control and also improves self-esteem. If possible, these approaches should be discussed and complemented together with friends and family. Envisioning coping strategies already applied to problematic situations and exploring further options leads to an increased awareness helpful when approaching difficult situations. Consequently, this supports and strengthens the individual's coping-ability (Kaluza2005; Lyubomirsky 2008). This is regarded to be particularly important for adolescents, as the coping-ability plays a central role during this phase of life (Seiffge-Krenke 2006).

Serenity.

The main strategy for enhancing *serenity* is a relaxation exercise. Progressive muscle relaxation (PMR) was chosen, as it is easy to learn and leads to a feeling of calm and balance. Furthermore, this strategy—if executed regularly—very quickly leads to first successes, which again influence the maintenance positively. The exercise designed for daily practice with an approximate duration estimate of 30 min, however it can be shorter at first. Optional combination of several modules corresponding with different body parts leaves this exercise very flexible with regard to its duration. It can also easily be applied to specific, potentially problematic body parts (Kaluza 2005).

Optimization.

The next strategy is designed to support the art-of-living-domain *optimization* . Students are asked to familiarize themselves with time management and its strategies using literature and the internet. They were provided with the links to relevant webpages. The techniques demonstrated there enable a more efficient time management (Seiwert1995).

Positive attitude towards life.

In order to support the art-of-living-domain *positive attitude towards life* the students take part in the happiness-beans-exercise. The participants are asked to put 5 beans or other objects of similar size into their right trouser pocket. Every time they experience a positive, pleasant or beautiful event, one bean is transferred from the right into the left. At the end of the day the beans in the left pocket are counted, while reminiscing about each respective moment. This exercise is designed to direct the participants' attention towards the bright side of life. Consequently, this leads to a more positive attitude towards life itself (Seligman 2004).

Self-efficacy.

The last strategy corresponds with the art-of-living-domain (perceived) *self-efficacy*. This is particularly important, as students with positive *self-efficacy* approach tasks in a more optimistic manner, difficulties and setbacks are perceived rather as challenges. Consequently, these students prove to be less nervous and more task-oriented. In order to support this domain, participants are asked to identify goals they want to achieve within the next week as well as factors that cause them to succeed. These factors are to be recalled frequently, until the objective is successfully achieved. Manifesting this mastery-experience increases the (perceived) self-efficacy (Schwarzer and Jerusalem 2002).

5.2.4 Results

5.2.4.1 Analyses of the Pretest-Posttest Comparisons

As a first step we performed an analysis of variance with repeated measurement with time (pretest-posttest) and group as independent variables. We were looking for group*time interactions. For the variables for which there were group*time interactions we calculated planned contrasts to test for which groups these interactions exist. Finally, we wanted to know whether there were training effects for the group with experimenter defined assignment of the art-of-living strategies (experimental group 3), because we know which strategies were trained in this group. Training effects were expected as changes for the trained strategies from pretest to posttest. Therefore, we performed t-tests for dependent variables for group 3 between pretest and posttests measures. Analyses of variance yielded group*time interaction for overall art-of-living $F(3,160) = 2{,}75$; $p < .05$; $\eta^2 = .05$. Subsequent analyses for art-of-living subscales yielded interaction effects (cf. Table 5.6) for *openness* and *positive attitude towards life*. For these variables which show a significant interaction effect we also perform subsequent contrast analyses, yielding for *overall art-of-living* (cf. Fig. 5.6) differences between control and experimental group 2, and similarly differences between control and experimental group 3, but not for differences between control and experimental group 1. Regarding *openness* we find (cf. Fig. 5.7) differences between control and experimental group 2, and similarly differences between control and experimental group 3, but not for differences between control and experimental group 1. With respect to *positive attitude towards life* there were differences between experimental group 2 and experimental group 1 and also between experimental group 3 and experimental group 1, cf. Fig. 5.8. For the comparisons of the means of pretest and posttest for the strategies assigned by the experimenter in group 3 we found significant effects for *overall art-of-living*, for *coping* and for *optimization* but not for *serenity*, *positive attitude towards life* and *self-efficacy*, cf. Table 5.7.

5.2.4.2 Analyses of the Diaries

To provide a sound data base for the diary data we combined the subjects from the three experimental groups only for students who worked on the diary for at least 12 days. Only a part of the participants answered the diary questions with this frequency. Therefore, these diary data are very interesting but are surely not representative and interpretations of these results have to be derived with caution.

We performed linear trend analysis (hypothesis 3) for the overall diary scale *art-of-living*. Results show that art-of-living develops positively over a fortnight (see Fig. 5.9). However, this trend is not significant: $F = 1.62$; $df1 = 1$; $df2 = 12$; $b0 = 3.13$; $b1 = .02$ n.s., that means art-of-living has at beginning a value of 3.13 and is increasing daily for .02 units.

Table 5.6 Significant results of analyses of variance and contrasts

Variable	Comparison	df1, df2	F	η^2
Art-of-living overall	All groups	3/160	2.75	.05
Openness	All groups	3/160	2.63	.05
Positive attitude towards life	All groups	3/160	3.57	.06
Art-of-living overall	Experimental group 2 versus control group	1/76	5.07	.06
Openness	Experimental group 2 versus control group	1/76	5.64	.07
Art-of-living overall	Experimental group 3 versus control group	1/83	5.14	.06
Openness	Experimental group 3 versus control group	1/83	5.94	.07
Positive attitude towards life	Experimental group 2 versus experimental group 1	1/77	7.61	.09

$p < .05$ for all tests

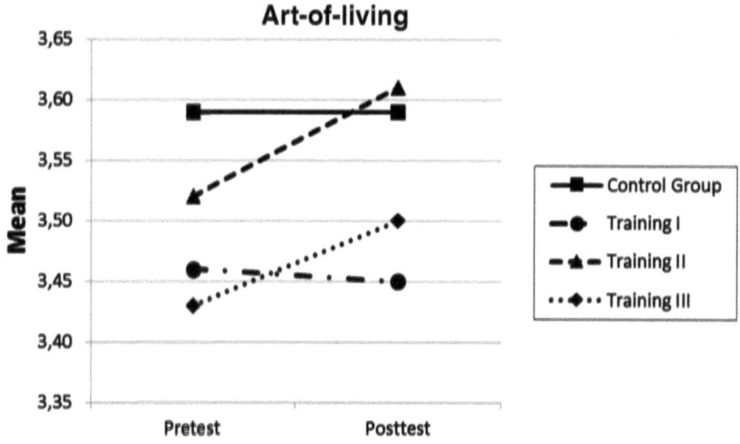

Fig. 5.6 Time × group interaction for *overall art-of-living*

Likewise, we also performed linear trend analysis for well-being. Results show that well-being is increasing during the observation period. This trend is significant (see Fig. 5.10), F = 6,24; df 1 = 1; df2 = 12; b0 = 3,23; b1 = .06; $p < .05$; that means well-being has at the beginning a value of 3.23 and is significantly increasing by .06 units each day. In sum, the diary data are sparse but show a non-significant increase for art-of-living and a significant trend for well-being.

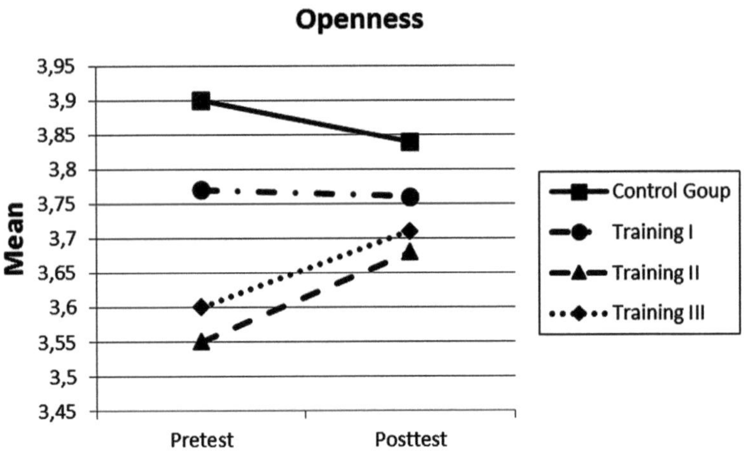

Fig. 5.7 Time × group interaction for the subscale *openness*

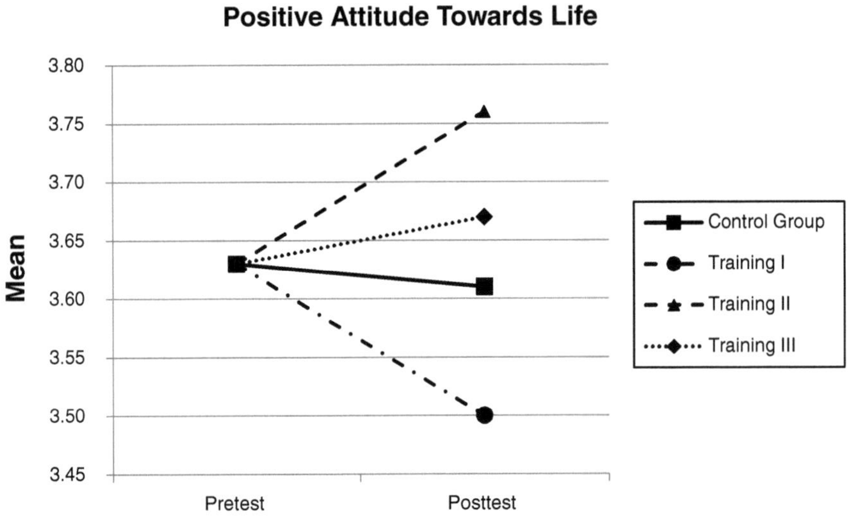

Fig. 5.8 Time × group interaction for the subscale *positive attitude towards life*

Table 5.7 Results of *t* test for pretest-posttest comparisons for group 3 where the strategies were assigned by the experimenter

Variable	df1, df2	F	η^2
Art-of-living overall	1/42	9.53*	.19
Coping	1/42	3.84*	.08
Serenity	1/42	0.57	–
Optimization	1/42	7.25*	.15
Positive attitude towards life	1/42	0.93	–
Self-efficacy	1/42	2.02	–

* $p < .05$

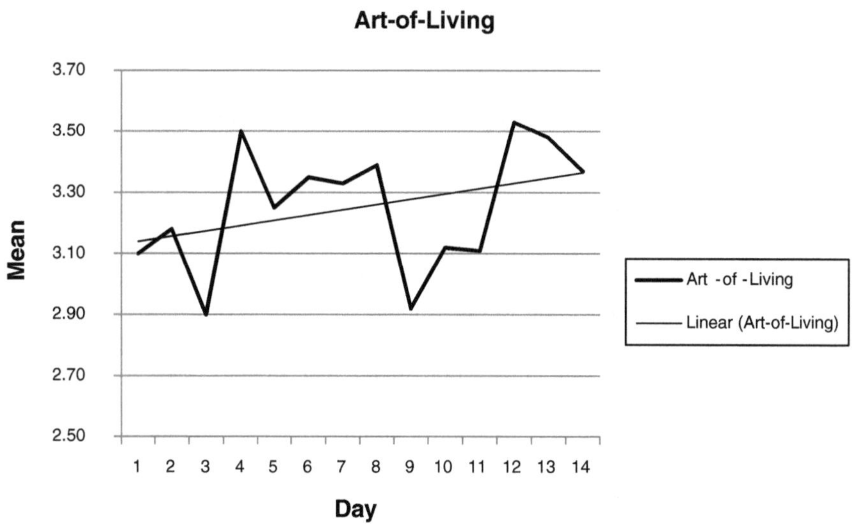

Fig. 5.9 Trend analysis for *overall art-of-living*

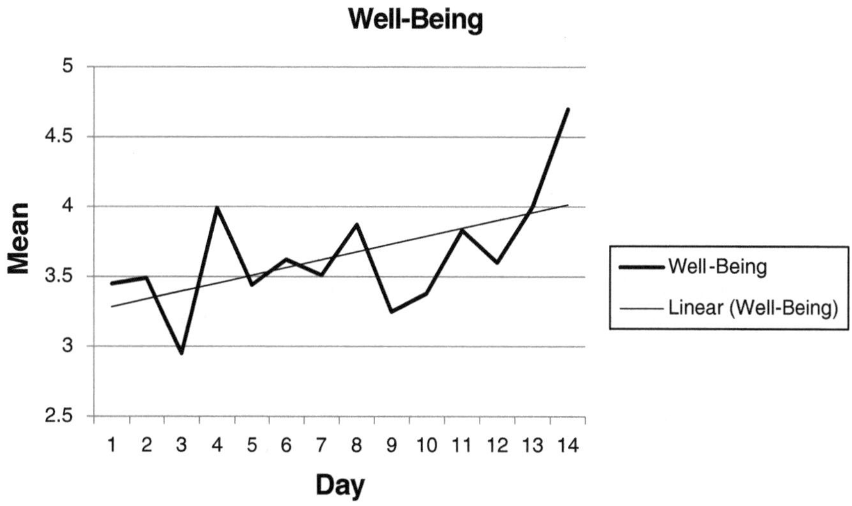

Fig. 5.10 Trend analysis for *well-being*

5.2.4.3 Choice of Strategies in the Autonomous Group 1

Experimental group 1 consisted of students who could choose among all art-of-living strategies which strategy they wanted to enhance. We wanted to know whether they applied strategies they were already familiar with or not. We compared information for an individual from one art-of-living pretest subscale with the other pretest subscale means which showed whether they applied a strategy often or seldom. If a value for a subscale was high compared to this mean (greater than: mean + half a standard deviation), we interpreted this as unsuitable: the subject has chosen a strategy which he already often applies; if the value was near the mean (greater than: mean − half a standard deviation and lower than: mean + half a standard deviation) we interpreted it as neutral and if it was clearly below the mean (lower than: mean − half a standard deviation) as suitable. This categorization follows the idea that a strategy is suitable to learn when it is not used very often. Because we had no data regarding real strategy use, we collected data using an extra sample which was comparable to our sample (N = 36, between 15 and 20 years old). We asked daily which strategy was applied. We compared the pretest information with this additional information about real strategy use. A comparison between the selected strategies (179 total) and the individual pretest results demonstrated that the students selected a strategy complementing their deficient scales only 45 times, while 47 times they selected a neutral one, whereas strategies corresponding with already highly developed scales were chosen 87 times. In sum, these results regarding to training group I show that students tend to choose strategies corresponding with their non-deficient art-of-living-domains.

5.2.5 *Discussion*

The assumption regarding the effectiveness of all training types could not be confirmed. For group I (the autonomous choice) there were no differences compared to the control group whereas training types II and III led to a significant increase in the art-of-living-scores measured directly after the training. Training type I appears to be less suitable for implementation when working with students. This is illustrated by the art-of-living-scores which do not significantly change over time when compared to the control group or any other experimental group. This result is reflected by the participants' choice of strategies. The students selected strategies corresponding with their non-deficient art-of-living-domains nearly twice as frequently as deficient strategies. A possible explanation for this could be the participants' expectations: Implementing the strategies they are already good at into their daily routine, the students expect a fast, significant effect. However, they will not learn very much for strategies they already know.

Regarding the diaries a significant linear trend could be observed for *well-being*. In sum, for this group of students enhancement of art-of-living by training seems to be possible. The best way for choosing art-of-living strategies seems to be deficit oriented that means, the recommendation would be to exercise strategies for which one is not good at the beginning and has the potential to improve.

5.2.5.1 Limitations and Future Research Opportunities

This study in a school context is affected by a series of problems which could occur in real life contexts. First, a follow-up test was planned but the data base was not sound enough for serious analyses. A large group of students did not want to answer a lot of questions again. Second, as could be seen, there were differences in the pretest values, which points to the problem, that the baseline for the groups might be different. But as Fig. 5.6 shows whereas one could argue that there might be a floor effect for the control group, this is essentially not true for the experimental group 1, for which there is much opportunity to enhance. Although there are already effects of the training the students complained that the training seemed too short for them. Compared to normal school topics the art-of-living contents were presented without much recapitulation. Also the lengthy test for art-of-living where criticized by the students. Therefore, there is the necessity to develop a shorter measurement instrument, especially for this group of participants.

The training should be both expanded and integrated further into the academic routine in order to enable more students to participate in art-of-living-trainings. Furthermore, one could think about inclusion of people in the training who could function as model or as assistants, e.g. parents and teachers (Seiffge-Krenke 2006; Gilman et al. 2009).

Moreover, art-of-living-strategies should be taught to younger students, supporting processes enabling optimism and self-efficacy earlier on. This is important, as these variables already begin to develop during childhood (Gilman et al. 2009).

5.2.5.2 Conclusion

Special kinds of art-of-living-trainings can increase *art-of-living* and *well-being*. The option of choosing the strategies has an influence on the training's effectivity, as the selection of suitable strategies is vital for an increase in the art-of-living-domains. In particular, strategies adapted to individual deficits and needs have a high potential for positive training effects.

5.3 Happiness at Work. A Training to Increase Art-of-Living at Work

Gesche Janzarik, Jessica Lang, Bernhard Schmitz

5.3.1 Introduction

People spend a big part of their lives at their working place. It is not surprising that the characteristics of a job are of particular importance for a person's well-being and satisfaction (Lopez et al. 2014). In this context the question arises whether satisfaction and psychological health only depend on external, job-related factors or whether the individual itself can contribute something to develop them. As can be seen in Sect. 3.8., we aimed at capturing the relationships between art-of-living and components of occupational success as well as self-fulfillment. With regard to the findings that there are high correlations we assume that working as a domain is an important aspect of art-of-living.

Research of Wrzesniewski et al. (1997) shows that every job principally has the potential to contribute to a person's happiness and satisfaction. According to that, it's not the predetermined task that decides about a person's satisfaction, much more it's the inner attitude of the person about his or her work that is the critical factor.

Berg et al. (2013) describe a similar approach in their job crafting model. Job crafting is the designing of the work by the employee himself by changing his task or the perception of his task in a way that makes him experience it as more interesting, meaningful and motivating which then leads to higher satisfaction, more motivation and better performance (Berg et al. 2013; Hackman and Oldham 1980; Grant 2007).

Under the assumption that people have an influence on their job satisfaction, how can people be supported to enhance their working life quality? In this study the main idea is to apply strategies and adapt attitudes belonging to the art-of-living concept. Which kind of strategies might be helpful? According to Diener (1984) the satisfaction with life is marked by the presence of positive and absence of negative emotions. The knowledge about the own feelings and the competence to regulate them, the ability to "perceive ones emotions and influence their intensity, duration and quality through cognition and behavior" (Lammers 2011, p. 49), can be seen as a fundamental of a positive attitude towards life which leads to a satisfied and fulfilled life. To have a good self-knowledge and to mindfully perceive the own emotions as well as strengths and weaknesses is central for a self-determined way of living and to find the meaning in the own life (Schmid 2007). Experiencing meaning sets free resources of the soul and mind (Schmid 2007). For example, Steger and Dik (2009) could prove that people which have a meaning in their life are more satisfied and optimistic.

In addition, dealing well with difficult situations and the conviction to cope with stressors and difficult requirements based on own abilities is also important for having a good and happy life. In this context, trainings of problem-solving skills can strengthen self-consciousness and locus of control and to become acquainted with methods to cope with future problems independently. While dealing with a personal straining situation is of interest to achieve good results to be open to new experiences and to act effectively as well as to feel serenely.

These and further results from research show that satisfaction and well-being of employees do not only depend on external factors predetermined by the task or the company. Much more does every person have the possibility to work on his own satisfaction. The philosophy of art-of-living describes a way of how to reach this (see Chap. 1). Art-of-living is related to measures of well-being and can be assigned to positive psychology. It deals with the conditions and processes that enable self-development of the individual. Art-of-living is based on several components. Strategies for all these components can be learned and therefore can be changed.

Based on this approach the current study developed a training especially tailored to the needs of working people in which they learn art-of-living strategies to actively improve their (working-) satisfaction. Additionally, it was assumed that also *resilience* can be effected by an art-of-living intervention. As can be seen in Chap. 3, Schmitz and Schmidt (2014) found out that there are correlations between the art-of-living and resilience. Regarding theoretical considerations and based on the definition of resilience (Baumgardner and Crothers 2010) a selection of some components of art-of-living has been made: *positive attitude towards life, coping, optimization, serenity, self-efficacy, openness, self-knowledge* and *self-determined way of living*. They were assumed to be important in the context of work. Tasks and strategies to train them were conducted.

5.3.2 Goals and Hypothesis

The fundamental goal of the study was the development, conduction and evaluation of a training to increase art-of-living. With the intervention art-of-living in the context of employment should be trained. The participants of the training were supposed to be enabled to develop individual art-of-living strategies which were especially tailored to the critical points in their personal working environment. The acquired skills should support them to make their private and professional daily life more satisfying and less stressful.

The following hypothesis were postulated:

1) The participation at the training causes a significant increase in the dependent variables whose related components were topic in the training, that means an increased value for the *art-of-living* scales *positive attitude towards life, coping, optimization, serenity, self-efficacy, openness, self-knowledge and self-determined way of living*. As a consequence we expect also effects for *satisfaction with life* and *resilience*.

2) The values of the dependent variables that show a significant increase after the training, do not decrease until follow up 4 weeks after the training but increase or stay at the level of the posttest.

5.3.3 Method

5.3.3.1 Design

The training focused on eight selected components of art-of-living as training contents: *positive attitude towards life, coping, self-knowledge, optimization, serenity, self-efficacy, openness* and *self-determined way of living*. The training consisted of four training units that took place at an interval of 1 week. Each of the four units lasted about 150 min. The participants of the experimental group (EG) took part in all four units. The control group (CG) only went through a first 60 min long training unit, the other three units followed after the end of the study.

The longitudinal data collection consisted of three measurement dates: a pretest (t1) before the first training unit, a posttest after the training (t2) and a follow-up 4 weeks after the last unit (t3).

5.3.3.2 Participants

The sample consisted of working people, who were on a monthly salary or worked as freelance employees for a company. The sample size was $N = 40$. The age ranged from 20 to 52 years ($M = 34.51$, $SD = 7.95$).

All in all six companies took part in the study. As it was not possible to randomize the employees of different companies in EG and CG due to organizational reason of the companies, a quasi-experimental design was used. The training units took place in the respective company. The groups consisted of five to eight participants. The small group size made it possible to pay attention to individual questions and problems.

5.3.3.3 Measures

Art-of-Living Questionnaire

The original questionnaire measuring the art-of-living by Schmitz and Schmidt (2014) was used (see Chap. 2). The Cronbach's α for the overall art-of-living in the present study amounts .94 for the three points of measurement (pretest, posttest and follow-up-test).

Resilience Scale (RS-11)

The Resilience Scale (Wagnild and Young 1993) correlates positively with the questionnaire measuring the art-of-living, s. Chap. 3 Table 3.9. It measures resilience. It consists eleven items, which are to be answered on a 7-point answer scale (from 1 = *strongly disagree* to 7 = *strongly agree*). The results of this study could show good internal consistencies: $\alpha = .91$ for pretest, $\alpha = .93$ for posttest and $\alpha = .94$ for follow-up-test.

Satisfaction with Life Scale (SWLS)

Previous research found out a high correlation between art-of living and satisfaction with life scale (see Chap. 2) by Scale Diener, Emmons, Larsen and Griffin, 1985 (in the German version of Glaesmer et al. 2011). The internal consistencies in the present study amounts to $\alpha = .81$ for the pretest, $\alpha = .75$ for the posttest and $\alpha = .80$ for the follow-up-test.

5.3.3.4 Procedure

The developed training is based on four training sessions, which are described in the following, cf. Table 5.8. At the beginning of the first unit, the accompanying learning diary is treated. In each session a break with a relaxation exercise was conducted after about 1.5 h to train the component *serenity*.

Session 1: Positive Attitude Towards Life, Coping and Self-Knowledge

The participants were at first asked to think about their past, about what distinguishes their lives, which highs and lows they had so far and where they see themselves now in their life. These thoughts should be visualized by a "life line" on a flipchart. The participants presented themselves by their "lifelines" to the other employees and to the trainer. Afterwards the trainer gave a short talk about the topic art-of-living and an overview about the structure of the training's contents.

The first exercise was based on the ABC-theory by Ellis (1994). The participants should recognize that not only the situation is critical for their emotions, but primarily their mental appraisal. To collect different emotions each participant wrote a "negative" emotion and its purpose on one card and a "positive" emotion and its purpose on another one. The cards were placed by the participants on a board. Afterwards the plenum discussed about it. The goal of the exercise was to raise consciousness for the fact that there are no pure "negative" emotions but that each

Table 5.8 Research design

Group	(t1)	Training				(t2)	(t3)
EG (n = 25)	Pretest	Unit 1	Unit 2	Unit 3	Unit 4	Posttest	Follow-up
CG (n = 15)	Pretest	Unit 1 abridged	–	–	–	Posttest	Follow-up

emotion has a positive effect and should be perceived. Anger, for example, can lead to the attempt to assert one's rights or grief can help to say goodbye to something important.

In the next exercise the participants dealt with how to influence negative thoughts and emotions. In a partner exercise they worked on cognitive strategies against mental traps and related negative emotions. Together they developed helpful thoughts against catastrophe thinking, thinking negatively, only thinking about themselves and thinking about errors. The task followed the theory of cognitive behavior therapy by Beck, that has the goal to identify the patient's dysfunctional cognitions, to question them and to develop alternative functional cognitions (see Beck et al. 1979).

The next step was about dealing with own negative thoughts and the development of adequate coping strategies. For this, the participants should think back to a situation of their past of which they believed they ran into a mental trap. Then they chose three questions from a catalogue of questions which helped them to transform their dysfunctional thoughts into functional ones. Examples were "What can I learn from this situation?", "What is more important in my life than this event?", "How will I think later, in a month or in a year about it?" or "What am I proud of?". The participants noted their answers and could retrospectively newly interpret the experienced situation.

Afterwards the participants were familiarized with the learning diary and the homework for the time until the next training unit. They got the task to write down one agreeable and one negative emotion every evening. In addition they should write down the thought that triggered the emotion. For disagreeable emotions they should also note how they dealt with it and whether they used a strategy to cope with it. This could be, like worked out in the training unit, appraisal-oriented strategies such as to reinterpret the situation with helpful questions. All other strategies should be noted as well, however, such as to distract oneself, go for a run, do oneself something good, etc.

As a relaxation task an exercise for mindful breathing modelled after Kabat-Zinn and Hanh (2009) was conducted. The participants should attentively perceive their own breath and the related bodily experiences. They were asked to repeat the task regularly in the following weeks and to write down in their learning diary how they could integrate the mindful breathing in their everyday lives.

Session 2: Coping, Openness and Self-Efficacy

The training unit began with a short presentation about the topic stress. The talk conveyed how stress occurs, which symptoms it can cause in people and in which cases stress can negatively influence health. After that the participants collected reasons for every-day stress at work and noted them on cards e.g. continuous availability, increased pressure at work, too little physical exercise, a too narrow schedule etc. Afterwards the results were discussed. In the course of the next exercise, the participants worked out useful thought pattern to counteract stress at work. Parts of the exercise were taken from the training manual about coping with stress by Kaluza (2005). Small groups were formed to work on a worksheet about one of the following five obstructive thought patterns and to present them to the plenum afterwards.

(A) *Be the very best!*—This thought pattern is about perfectionist performance and an exaggerated demand on the completion of tasks.

(B) *Be recognized by all!*—This thought pattern mirrors the wish for recognition and social acceptance. It is about the exaggerated attempt to be liked by everybody and to avoid being criticized.

(C) *Stay totally independent!*—Behind this thought pattern is the wish to be personally independent and very much self-determined. The exaggerated striving for autonomy and the avoidance of dependences can in the long run lead to strain and overwork.

(D) *Be careful and stay always in control!*—This thought pattern reflects the need for control and safety. People who tend to it try to avoid the loss of control at any price and have difficulties to make decisions and take risks.

(E) *Go easy and avoid all negative things!*—People who tend to this thought pattern have learned early in life that it is better to avoid difficulties and effort. A reason for this is frequently a lack of trust in the own competences.

In the next step every participant chose an *obstructive* thought pattern that is typical for them and rephrased it as a *useful* thought pattern (e.g. "I want to disappoint my colleagues on no account" was rephrased as "I also think of myself, not everybody has to like me"). The participants were supposed to collect strategies how to internalize the new thought patterns to give up the automatic thought habits of years.

In the next exercise the participants were given simple techniques and ideas to make their every-day life less stressful and to improve their self-organization. For this, every participant could choose a method and work out its essential points with a worksheet to present them to the group afterwards. The applicability as well as the advantages and disadvantages of the single methods were discussed. The following techniques could be selected: the ABC-analysis, the ALPEN-method, the Eisenhower-principle, the performance curve, the Pareto-principle, the concept of the silent hour as well as the Mind-Map-Method (for a more detailed description see Seiwert 2014), additionally the thought-stop-method (Landmann and Schmitz 2007) and the method of the SMART-objective.

On the basis of the stressors collected at the beginning of the training unit it was examined which technique could defuse which stressor. Afterwards the participants could present their own strategies to reduce their stress at work. Every participant chose at least two of the newly learned methods that fit his personal professional life. As a homework they should deal with the strategies more closely and integrate them in their every-day life.

As relaxation exercise of the second training unit a mindfulness exercise was conducted. For this, the trainer had brought several types of tea. The exercise was to perceive the hot tea with all senses and to enjoy the present moment preferably without zoning out or judging the situation mentally. The homework was to have a

5-min tea or coffee break every day until the next unit while practicing the principle of mindfulness.

Session 3: Self-Knowledge, Self-Determined Way of Living and Positive Attitude Towards Life

The training of problem-solving of the third training unit was done after the approach of D'Zurilla and Goldfried (1971) who distinguish between five steps to the solution of a problem: general problem-orientation, description of a problem, creation of alternative solutions, decision for one solution as well as action and evaluation.

At the beginning of the training unit the participants chose a part of their life which presented a stressor. It could for example be job-related stressors, such as common time pressure or nervousness due to an upcoming interview, social stressors such as interpersonal conflicts or also more complex problematic situations. With the help of a worksheet the participants described the chosen situation as precise as possible. If necessary the problem could be subdivided into smaller parts. Additionally the desired target state of the situation should be defined. Afterwards every participant got a flipchart paper to clearly portray the situation for the other participants. The posters were hung up in the room. Every participant presented his problem to the group and answered their questions.

In a second step, the participants noted their own suggestions for solving the problem in their transfer diary. Afterwards every participant got a pile of post-its. A creative brain storming was conducted in which they created possible solutions for each other's problems. On every post-it an idea was written before they were glued to the posters. The goal was to develop as many different solutions for one problem as possible. Afterwards the participants could ask questions about the ideas of the others and discuss advantages and disadvantages.

In a third step the participants noted the newly learned possibilities to solve the problem on their worksheets and chose the one that would most probably lead to success in their opinion.

In a fourth step the realization of the solution should be planned. For this, the participants developed a formulation of the goal that was as realistic, precise and close to behavior as possible. The solution should be decomposed in precise single steps if necessary. Reflecting possible difficulties also belonged to planning.

The fifth step, putting of the written plan into practice, should be realized as the participant's homework. To facilitate the transfer and to increase locus of control, a mental imagination task was conducted. The participants were supposed to relax through the method of mindful breathing and were then instructed to imagine their problematic situation and how they mastered them in the way they had targeted.

The relaxation followed the method of progressive relaxation by Jacobson (2011). The scientifically acknowledged procedure is an easily learned relaxation method where one can reach a state of relaxation of the whole body by consciously contracting and relaxing certain muscle groups. The exercise should be conducted at least five times until the next unit. In that process the participants should write down in their transfer diary how the repeated practicing influenced their perception of stress.

Session 4: Self-Knowledge

In the last training unit the participants should deal with their own traits and strengths. For this, they filled in the worksheets of the session at home before the unit. With a semantic differential (e.g. taciturn—talkative) (cf. Osgood 1964) they judged themselves as well as anonymously all other participating colleagues. Furthermore, they chose five strengths from a list of 38 that fitted to them best. Own, not listed strengths could also be noted. The choice of the 38 strengths consisted for one thing of the character strengths of the Values in Action Inventory of Strengths (VIA-IS) by Peterson and Seligman (2004), for another of the talents of the classification of strengths of the Gallup Organization (see Buckingham and Clifton 2001). Apart from judging their strengths, the participants should also chose three strengths of their participating colleagues and write down reasons for their choice. Self- and peer-assessments were scanned and send to the trainers via e-mail. The homework also included questions about reflection: In which private/professional situations do I use my strengths? What am I especially proud of? Where are my weaknesses? Which traits do I want to develop and which do I want to display less often?

In the first part of the training unit the participants got the results from the self- and peer-assessment. They could judge by the sematic differential in what way the own judgment differed from the mean of the peer assessment. The participants were supposed to become aware of their outward effect. Additionally they got a written feedback about which strengths the other participants attributed to them. The exercise's goal was to broaden the own self-image in a positive way.

In the second part the participants dealt with their own lifestyle. The exercise followed Wengenroth (2012). The participants evaluated their different areas of life in individual work, on the one hand according to their importance, on the other hand according to how much time and energy they invested in this area. The goal was to reflect the own life situation and to find differences between their lifestyle and their aspirations. Then, the participants choose two areas which they did not pay enough attention to even although they were of high importance to them. They wrote down how these areas should ideally be designed and planed specific steps to enforce these areas in their lives. Furthermore, they reflected which obstacles could be in their way.

In the last part of the training the participants found access to the topic search for meaning in a creative way. They got the task to express their life in a piece of art. For this, magazines with pictures and other handicraft materials were handed out. The following questions should be examined: What are my professional and private goals for the future? What is important to me? What shall my life stand for? In which direction do I want to go? Which values shall characterize my life?

Instead of a relaxation task, a thankfulness task (following Berking 2008) was conducted in the last training unit. The exercise was again initiated by mindful breathing. Subsequently, the participants were supposed to remember in a relaxed and mindful state all the positive things that happened in their lives and how much better they were off in comparison to some other people in the world. Afterwards the participants wrote down what they are thankful for in life. The goal of the exercise was to perceive and acknowledge the positive aspects in life.

Diary for the Support of Transfer into Daily Life

In the course of the training a diary (Schmitz and Perels 2011) was used. It comprises the content of the various exercises, the tasks that should be worked on between units as well as questions about reflection and objective.

By the use of the transfer-support diary the process of reflection should be deepened and the training success should be supported. Many studies prove that it could be sufficient just to observe one's own behavior can lead to a change of behavior in the desired way (e.g. Korotitsch and Nelson Gray 1999). Since the participants had the possibility to write down personal thoughts, emotions and problems in the diary, it was only the participants' responsibility to fill it in and was not checked by the trainers to ensure privacy.

5.3.4 *Results*

To test the postulated hypotheses a repeated measures multivariate analysis of variance was conducted. It was investigated whether differences in the means of the different times of measurement were caused by membership to one of the groups (experimental group, control group). The dependent variables were the subscales of the art-of-living questionnaire, s*atisfaction with life* and *resilience*. Afterwards, it was tested with pairwise t-tests whether the increase of the means in the experimental group from the first to the second time of measurement or from the second to the third was significant.

5.3.4.1 Testing of Hypothesis 1

The results of the MANOVA are listed in Table 5.9. A significant time × group interaction was found for the component *positive attitude towards life*, $F(2, 76) = 3.35$, $p = .040$, $\eta^2 = .081$ (Fig. 5.11). The results of the post-hoc analyses are listed in Table 5.10. The differences between the means of pre- and post-test for the experimental group was not significant.

For *coping* a significant time × group interaction could be found as well, $F(2, 76) = 13.56$, $p < .001$, $\eta^2 = .263$ (Fig. 5.12). The results of the t-test showed that

Table 5.9 Multivariate analyses of variance

Scales	F	df	η^2
Balance	0.09	2/76	.002
Coping	13.56***	2/76	.263
Serenity	3.16*	2/76	.077
Savoring	0.29	2/76	.008
Shaping of living conditions	0.82	2/76	.021
Physical care	0.44	2/76	.011
Openness	0.98	2/76	.025
Optimization	0.14	2/76	.004
Positive attitude towards life	3.35*	2/76	.081
Self-determined way of living	0.75	2/76	.019
Self-knowledge	8.01***	2/76	.174
Self-efficacy	2.94	2/76	.072
Social contact	1.32	2/76	.034
Integrating different areas of living	0.58	2/76	.015
Art-of-living	1.85	2/76	.047
Satisfaction with life	2.24	2/76	.056
Resilience	7.52***	2/76	.165

η^2 = partial eta squared
* $p \leq .05$; ** $p \leq .01$; *** $p \leq .001$

the increase in the mean from pre- to post-test for the experimental group was significant, $t(24) = -6.18$, $p < .001$, but not for the control group.

A further significant time × group interaction was found for *serenity*, $F(2, 76) = 3.16$, $p = .048$, $\eta^2 = .077$ (Fig. 5.13). The post-hoc analyses from pre- to post-test showed a significant increase in the mean of the experimental group, $t(24) = -2.39$, $p = .025$, but not for the control group.

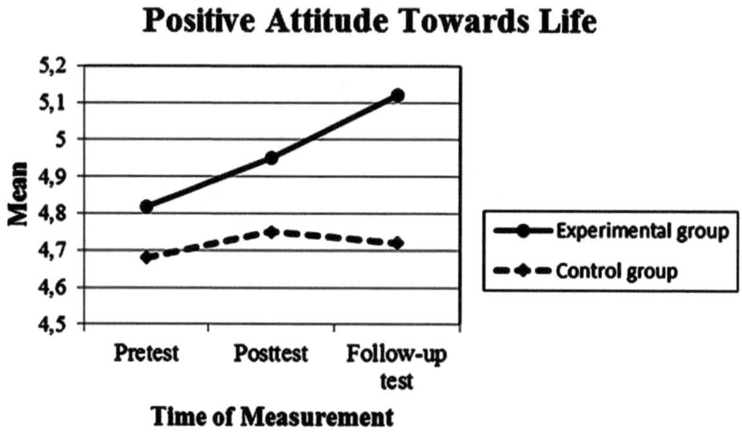

Fig. 5.11 Time × group interaction for the scale *positive attitude towards life*

Table 5.10 Post hoc analysis to test the differences between pre- and posttest for the experimental group and for the control group

Scales	Control group		Experimental group	
	t	df	*t*	*df*
Balance	−0.46	14	−0.58	24
Coping	0.00	14	−6.18***	24
Serenity	0.00	14	−2.39*	24
Savoring	0.67	14	−0.54	24
Shaping of living conditions	−0.31	14	−1.00	24
Physical care	−0.78	14	1.20	24
Openness	−1.07	14	1.42	24
Optimization	−1.12	14	−0.32	24
Positive attitude towards life	−0.85	14	−1.95	24
Self-determined way of living	−0.61	14	1.54	24
Self-knowledge	−0.64	14	−2.31*	24
Self-efficacy	0.72	14	−2.51*	24
Social contact	−1.68	14	0.86	24
Integrating different areas of living	0.00	14	−0.54	24
Art-of-living	−0.83	14	−1.20	24
Satisfaction with life	0.11	14	−0.50	24
Resilience	0.77	14	−5.36***	24

η^2 = partial eta squared
$^{*}p \leq .05$; $^{**}p \leq .01$; $^{***}p \leq .001$

A significant time × group interaction proved for *self-knowledge* as well, $F(2, 76) = 8.01$, $p = .001$, $\eta^2 = .174$ (Fig. 5.14). For the experimental group the subsequent t-test showed a significant increase from pre- to post-test, $t(24) = -2.31$, $p = .030$, but not for the control group.

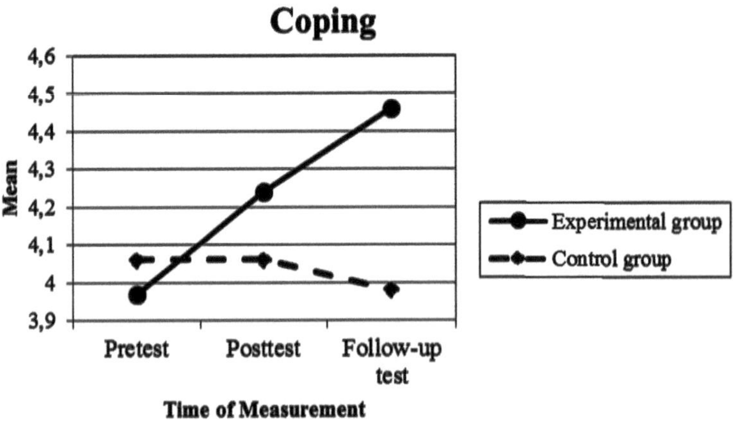

Fig. 5.12 Time × group interaction for the scale *coping*

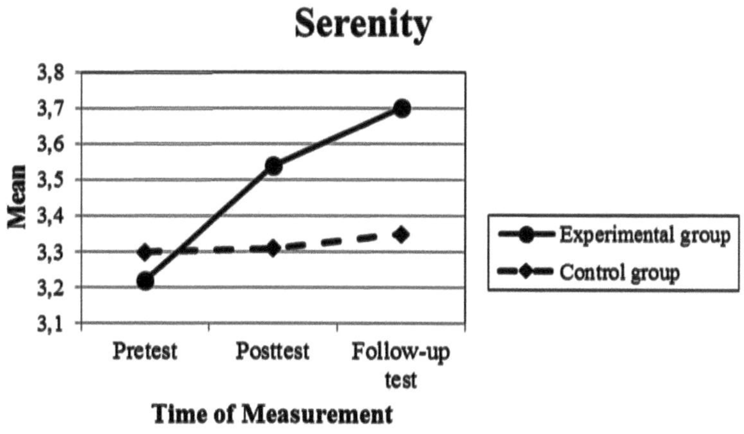

Fig. 5.13 Time × group interaction for the scale *serenity*

Additionally a significant time × group interaction could be found for the dependent variable *resilience*, $F(2, 76) = 7.52$, $p = .001$, $\eta^2 = .165$ (Fig. 5.15). The post-hoc analysis from pre- to post-test showed a significant increase in the mean for the experimental group, $t(24) = -5.36$, $p < .001$, but not for the control group.

For the subscales of the art-of-living questionnaire *optimization, self-efficacy, openness* and *self-determined way of living* and for the *satisfaction with life* no significant time × group interactions could be found. The post-hoc analyses for the control group were not significant in any of the subscales, cf. table 5.10.

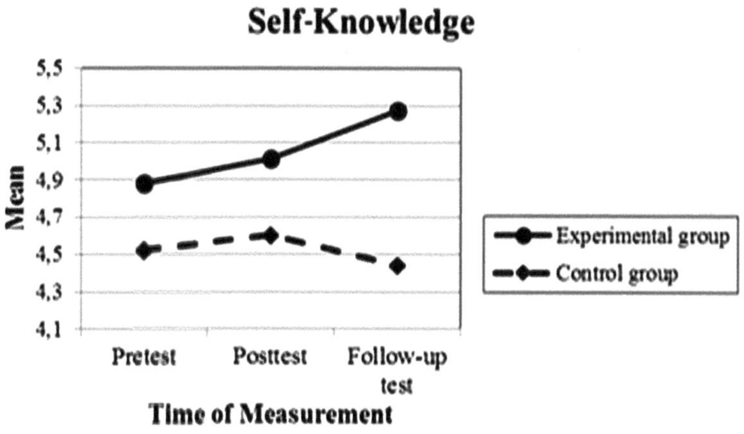

Fig. 5.14 Time × group interaction for the scale *self-knowledge*

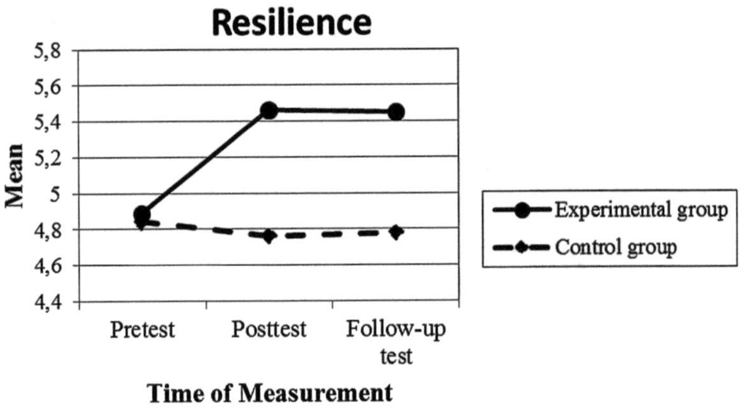

Fig. 5.15 Time × group interaction for the dependent variable *resilience*

5.3.4.2 Testing of Hypothesis 2

The results of all t-tests can be seen in Table 5.11 for the experimental group. The analyses could show that the means of the scales *coping, t*

Table 5.11 Post hoc analysis to test the differences between posttest and follow up test for the experimental group and for the control group

Scales	Control group		Experimental group	
	T	df	*t*	*df*
Balance	−0.76	14	0.25	24
Coping	0.86	14	−3.36**	24
Serenity	−0.30	14	−1.74	24
Savoring	−1.20	14	−0.69	24
Shaping of living conditions	0.38	14	−1.05	24
Physical care	−0.79	14	−1.23	24
Openness	−0.24	14	−0.99	24
Optimization	1.00	14	0.11	24
Positive attitude towards life	0.34	14	−3.62**	24
Self-determined way of living	0.44	14	−0.42	24
Self-knowledge	1.18	14	−4.26**	24
Self-efficacy	−2.45*	14	−2.04	24
Social contact	0.75	14	−0.91	24
Integrating different areas of living	−0.37	14	−1.74	24
Art-of-living	−0.01	14	−2.00	24
Satisfaction with life	0.77	14	−1.92	24
Resilience	−0.12	14	0.10	24

η^2 = partial eta squared
* $p \leq .05$, ** $p \leq .01$, *** $p \leq .001$

(24) = −3.36, $p = .003$, *self-knowledge* $t(24) = -4.26$, $p < .001$ and *positive attitude towards life*, $t(24) = -3.62$, $p = .001$, improved significantly from the second to the third time of measurement. For the scales *serenity*, $t(24) = -1.74$, $p = .094$ and *resilience*, $t(24) = 0.10$, $p = .920$, no significant differences were found, the means were stable from posttest to follow up. The control group showed only one change.

5.3.5 Discussion

5.3.5.1 The Effect of Training

The intervention influences some areas of art-of-living in a positive way. The results for the first hypothesis show that especially the abilities to deal with difficult situations and stress had improved. Comparing the results of the first and the second time of measurement, a significant improvement of the values for the scales *coping*, *serenity* and *self-knowledge* and *resilience* can be found. Other areas of art-of-living were possibly not examined enough by the intervention. As can be seen by the structure of the training, certain art-of-living competences were only trained in one session. Others, however, were trained more often or in a more intensive way. The scales *optimization, openness, self-efficacy and self-determined way of living* only found application in one unit. That might have caused the participants to deal too little with the respective art-of-living strategies and has therefore not resulted in a significant increase from pre- to post-test. In addition it cannot be assumed that the ability of self-determination can be learned from one day to the next. Schmid (2007) talks about a process that firstly requires the freeing of oneself from rules, norms and values directed by others, and then subsequently involves setting own goals, recognizing possibilities, living own values and finally finding personal meaning. Self-esteem "grows in time, needs patience and a long-term perspective as well" (Schmid 2007, p. 115), which can explain why the scales *self-efficacy* and *self-determined way of living* had not improved through a single training. Related to this self-determination process is the ability of self-knowledge (Schmid 2007), which could already be improved successfully through the training. When conceptualizing an intervention for art-of-living it should be paid attention to designing the unit and exercises in a way that is explicitly focused on certain art-of-living competences. The different areas of art-of-living should be treated with sufficient intensity and at best repeatedly to reach significant improvements. Interpreting the results of the current study it should also be taken into account that the training was primarily focused on the working context. Although Diener and Lucas (1999) found a correlation of .40 between job satisfaction and happiness in general, it can be assumed that the contents of the training were focused too specifically on work and that the life as such was treated too little.

Many of the contents were designed in a way that was chiefly applicable in the working context and improved the job satisfaction of the participants. The participants might not have been able to apply the contents to a broader context, especially since the questionnaire was filled in during work at the working place. Schwarz and Strack (1999) stress that the judgment of subjective well-being does not necessarily reflect a stable state. Much more important is the judgment about the own satisfaction made on the basis of information that are accessible at that time. It is possible that filling in the questionnaire during (stressing) tasks at work is not the optimal context.

5.3.5.2 Results of the Follow-Up

Looking at the difference of the means between the second and the third time of measurement, it can be seen that the values for the scales *coping*, *self-knowledge* and *positive attitude towards life* increased again. The values of the scales *serenity* and *resilience* showed no significant differences between posttest and follow-up. Therefore, the second hypothesis could be confirmed. The results make it clear that the increase of the values through the training is no short-term effect which vanishes after the intervention. For how long the increase of competence in these areas persists cannot be shown by the current design and will have to be examined in a future study.

5.3.5.3 Limitations of the Study

As already described, some areas of art-of-living were not dealt with intensively enough in the intervention. To be able to improve further areas, the training should last for a longer time and consist of more training units. An extension of the training to a longer program with about ten sessions could be considered. An accompanying standardized diary could be developed which is filled in regularly by the participants and which can be analyzed statistically afterwards. With the gained process data more precise findings about the course of the increase in art-of-living competences could be reached and individual training units could be improved specifically.

A further point of discussion is the size and make-up of the sample: only a sample of $N = 40$ could be reached. For this size a comparison between the training groups from the different companies was not reasonable. An interesting research subject would be the question whether work-related factors such as branch, working experience or certain tasks at work have an influence on learning art-of-living.

The participation at the training was voluntary for the individual employees. They agreed to be present at the four training units during working time and to fill in the questionnaire completely for all times of measurement. It can be assumed that the willingness for this additional effort crucially depends on the interest in the topic art-of-living, the motivation and the personal initiative of the employee. The meta-analysis of Bolier et al. (2013) deals with differences between self-selected and not-self-selected samples. Klauer and Leutner (2007) consider a sufficient degree of motivation as necessary requirement to initiate a successful learning process. It could be possible that the effects at hand were influenced to a certain degree by the motivation and openness of the participants. The results of the meta-analyses of Sin and Lyubomirsky (2009) confirm an effect of self-selection. The learning success could be smaller for a participation prescribed by the employer.

Especially from the point of view of the employer it can be interesting which influence the increase of art-of-living has on aspects such as job satisfaction and motivation of employees. Therefore, future research about art-of-living in the context of employment should use standardized instruments of organizational psychology, cf. Sect. 3.8. as well.

5.3.5.4 Conclusion

Whoever deals with questions about deliberate lifestyle should not ignore working life as a central part. The job does not only have an important standing with regard to the lifetime we invest in it. It can serve as a basis of satisfaction, can give meaning to life and influence the personal development in a crucial way.

Through the training the participants could gain more calmness. They developed a more positive attitude towards life, became conscious of their own values, strengths and attitudes and proved more robust against stress. When art-of-living can be trained as entire construct it means an important contribution to the life of employees. With regard to current problems of the business world such as an increasing numbers of sick days or lacking motivation of the employees it also presents an added value for the company behind it. These reflections show the high importance that an improvement of the abilities of art-of-living has for individuals and organizations.

5.4 A Web-Based Adaptive Training for the Art-of-Living

Janina Linten

5.4.1 Introduction

In this chapter we will describe ways to enhance art-of-living and well-being. In previous interventions a trainer instructed participants how to apply strategies of art-of-living. We could show that this way of delivering the training is effective. Because participants have to invest time to take part at trainings, it would be good, if the organization of the training context would support participation. If participants could choose themselves the place and time to deal with the exercises belonging to the training it would allow much more flexibility for attending such trainings.

Hence, the internet as a platform provides a great opportunity for such trainings. Online interventions enable participants to access and execute their training whenever they are able to do so. In addition, potential inhibitions are lowered, as subjects can remain mostly anonymous. However, this anonymity can cause a lack of motivation, since an explicit control authority is unavailable. Moreover, not all participants are sufficiently familiar with using the internet. An online training's further advantages include the option of adapting the training to individual needs as well as an incredibly more extensive outreach at very low costs (Manthey et al. 2014).

Manthey et al. (2014) proved that subjective well-being can be enhanced using cognitive exercises (e.g. describing the best possible self and letter of gratitude). The effect could still be measured 4 weeks after the intervention. The exercises were provided by downloadable work sheets as well as by video-instructions (Manthey et al. 2014).

Another online study focused on emotional self-regulation, the relationship with oneself as well as the sleep quality (Murray et al. 2015). In this study, the authors used exercises from the Acceptance and Commitment Therapy (ACT) as well as the Mindfulness-Based Cognitive Therapy (MBCT). The 3-week training comprised the elements *clarifying goals, self-acceptance, developing mindfulness* as well as *identifying goals* (as a guideline for future actions). The results showed that mindfulness-interventions can be realized online, effectively and significantly enhancing the Quality of Life (QoL, Murray et al. 2015).

Developing an online training for the art-of-living was the aim of the present study. The selection of contents was supposed to be based on the results of the study mentioned above. It can be inferred from Gräfe and Schmitz (Sect. 5.2) that enabling participants to choose art-of-living-strategies does not lead to an optimal assignment. Instead direct assignment by the experimenter or strategy-selection based on deficient art-of-living-domains proved to produce significantly better results. In the present study an approach integrating both assignment alternatives was used. The art-of-living-strategies least used by participants within a prestudy were applied. Based on these research findings a training was developed. This prestudy measured 110 participants' respective scores for the art-of-living-subscales *balance, coping, serenity, savoring, shaping of living conditions, physical care, openness, optimization, positive attitude towards life, reflection, self-actualization, self-knowledge, self-determined way of living, self-efficacy, meaning, social contact* and *integrating different areas of living* (see Chap. 2. revised edition.). Lower scores were found for *serenity, physical self-care, optimization* and *self-efficacy.*

Consequently, a training designed to enhance these competencies was designed. However, it was another important objective to influence art-of-living as a whole. Because we assume that the strategies of art-of-living have an effect on *satisfaction with life*, we suppose that *well-being* should increase as well.

5.4.2 Hypotheses

(1) The online training enhances *art-of-living* as well as *well-being*.
(2) The trainings effect persists when tested in a follow up study.

5.4.3 Method

Subjects assigned themselves to one of two groups depending on the time-periods which fitted best to their individual time schedule. The experimenter randomly determined which group performed as control- and which as experimental-group. The control-group was subjected to exactly the same training as the experimental-group, only at a later point in time (see Table 5.12). The training was provided using the open-source platform *Moodle* (see Fig. 5.16). The exercises were explained via videos (GoAnimate) and written instructions.

Each video and each instruction followed a common theme. The videos should on one hand explain the exercises clearly and on the other hand present scientific findings about or advantages of an exercise (to create motivation). The explanation of the exercise was made with key points and in the form of different questions. This should give an intuitive approach to the exercises. For nearly every exercise a video was made, only very short exercises or those not considered practical for video-presentation were described with written instructions.

5.4.3.1 Participants

The training was conducted and evaluated using the data of a sample of $N_1 = 65$ participants with a mean age of $M = 37$ ($SD = 11.79$). Participants can be characterized by their respective relationship status (35 % single, 60 % in a relationship), profession (32 % students, 29 % (un)securely employed) and parenthood (55 % none, 45 % 1–3 children). Before and after the online training a pre- and post-test were conducted. Additionally the data required for the follow-up was measured 30 days later. $N_2 = 44$ people submitted their data.

Table 5.12 Design of the intervention study

Group	Pretest	Training	Posttest	Bonus exercises	Follow-up	Training
EG $N_1 = 26$ $N_2 = 18$	Questionnaires	Online-training, three weeks	Questionnaires	Optional bonus exercises	Questionnaires	
CG $N_1 = 26$ $N_2 = 18$				Four weeks		Online-training, 3 weeks

N_1 = number of subjects who took part at two times of measurement (Pre/Post); N_2 = number of subjects who took part at three times of measurement; EG = experimental group, CG = control group

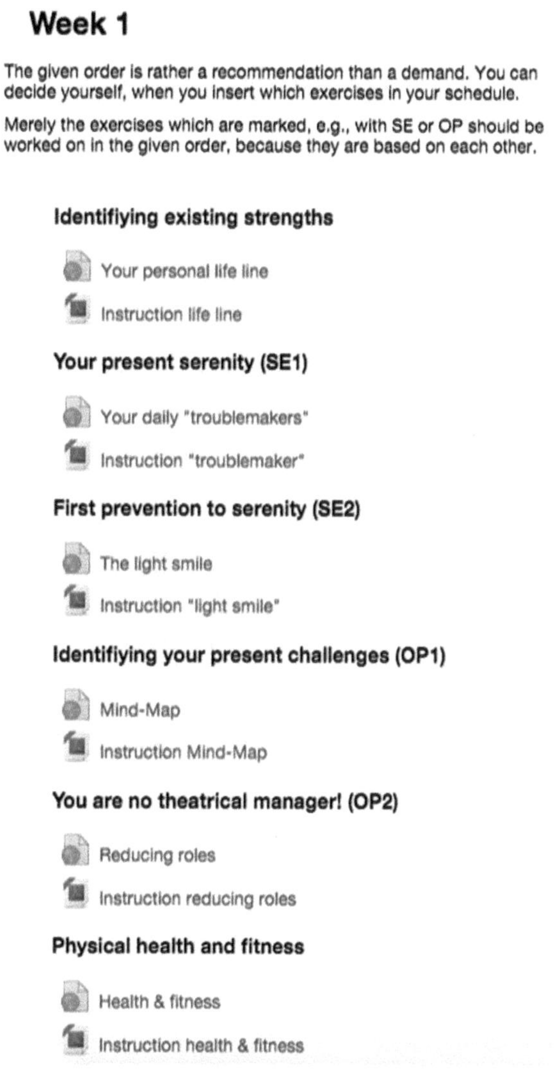

Fig. 5.16 Homepage of the course in Moodle

5.4.3.2 Measures

Art-of-Living

The *overall art-of-living* was determined using the questionnaire's abridged version (see Sect. 2.4, $\alpha = .93^2$).

[2]Reliabilities were calculated in the course of this study.

Subjective well-being

In order to measure the *satisfaction with life* the satisfaction with life scale ($\alpha = .89$[1]) was used, cf. Chap. 2.

5.4.3.3 Procedure

The training was divided in three units which were conducted in a weekly sequence.

- *Identifying of the current state and the target state* (week 1)
- *What can I change specifically? What could help me? What could inhibit me?* (week 2)
- *What do I do specifically from today on and how?* (week 3)

The aim was also an active work on the developed subgoals.

According to this scheme as well as to the solution- and resources-oriented view the training's contents were conceptualized. The goal was that every participant could find out for himself what he wishes for, what is already going smoothly and what is improvable. For this it is especially important to formulate questions and instructions in a way that enables the participants to identify as many of their resources as possible and to derive an active competence to act. It follows the theory that something can only be changed when a precise picture of the goal is envisioned after the exploration of the current state and the person concerned is aware of their resources and possible actions. When the picture and the possible actions are envisioned in detail, the resulting motivation and anticipation can be helpful for developing the first approaches to act. This motivation also helps with the exercises which are to be applied immediately. It was the goal of the third week to strengthen certain contents and exercises even more. The detailed considerations of the past weeks should lead to specific impulses to act.

Welcoming Video

The training started with a video that explained the contents and the procedure of the training (see *conceptualization of the training*) and was supposed to increase the motivation for and the joy of the training. The concept of art-of-living was presented. Afterwards a further video followed to stress the advantages of writing down thoughts or insights.

Conclusion Video

The conclusion video served as repetition of the training's contents. It should stimulate a final reflection and refresh contents. Moreover, the individual exercises of the week could be transferred specifically to the individual contents of the training (*serenity, physical health and fitness, optimizing of time management, self-efficacy and self-knowledge conveyed by trusting in ones strengths*) and associated

Table 5.13 Overview of the exercises, sorted in order of appearance

Exercise (art-of-living sub-component)	Duration	Goal	Short description
Week 1			
Self-efficacy			
Your personal life-line	50 min	Identifying strengths and resources	Identifying positive experiences and mastered challenges
Serenity			
Your daily troublemakers	40 min	Dealing with the own serenity; transferring the gained insights to specific situations	Identifying the current state and visualizing the future
Self-efficacy and serenity			
The easy smile	2 min/day	Strengthening self-efficacy; facilitates an easy introduction to the training; leads over to preventive measures;	Early morning smile with triple breath; personally formulated daily successes
Optimization			
Mind-Map: Your personal time requirements	25 min	Discovering focuses, priorities and urge to change	Easy and motivating introduction through graphical approach, identifying the current state of the daily demands
Reduce roles	20 min	Setting temporal emphasis and priorities	Reducing roles in the daily life
Physical self-care			
Health and Fitness	20 min	Developing specific goals to promote motivation for a lasting physical self-care in the every-day life	"Assuming that your physical care just looks like it is optimum for you?"; mindfulness in context nutrition
Week 2			
Physical self-care, serenity and optimization			
Going to bed ritual	5–10 min	Increasing relaxation; better physical energy level	Establishing a going to bed ritual
Optimization			
The Eisenhower-principle	30 min	Learning a long-term method for the every-day life	Quick structuring of activities according to "importance" and "urgency" (A/B/C-tasks)

(continued)

Table 5.13 (continued)

Exercise (art-of-living sub-component)	Duration	Goal	Short description
Serenity			
Prevention for serenity	About 15 min	Preventive mindfulness to promote serenity permanently and implement it with little expenditure of time	PMR/Yoga/Mediation
Physical self-care			
Health and fitness in every-day life?	20 min + 15 min	Incentive for the first small step to promote motivation and facilitate the introduction to physical exercise	How can a determined goal be reached and which obstacles can be considered in advance
Self-efficacy			
Your future life-line 1: desired me	35 min	Envisioning picture of goal without everyday limits, promotion of motivation for target achievement	Generating own wishes for future
Your future life-line 2: The next 5 years	Included in time of exercise 1	Promotion of an attitude towards an independent designing of the future; identified resources from the life-line so far (week 1) strengthen self-confidence	Transfer aims on the close future; first step should be generated
Week 3			
Self-efficacy			
Your personal well-being diary	10 min, 15–20 min with supp.	Achievements of the day are perceived more strongly; promotion of mindfulness in the every-day life	Instead of negative daily events, positive ones should be remembered
Optimization			
"Disrupting time curve"	15 min	Identifying disruptions and planned use of the learned A/B/C tasks from the exercise about the Eisenhower principle	Temporal division and dynamics of the day
Silent hour	20 min	Clarification of the time lost through distractions	Planning of a daily appointment during which important tasks can be carried out without external stimuli

(continued)

Table 5.13 (continued)

Exercise (art-of-living sub-component)	Duration	Goal	Short description
Serenity			
Radical acceptance	–	Changing the attitude about stressful situations	Accept occurrences which cannot be influenced
Physical care			
Your deliberate cooking experience	30 min	The cooking experience should be used for relaxation and balancing, deliberate nutrition should be promoted	Mindfully chosen food (week 1) is to be prepared mindfully
Optimization			
Saying no (voluntary)	–	Motivation is raised and impulses to act are given—thereby better time management	Benefits of saying no is stressed
Optimization		Bonus exercises	
Fighting thieves of time	20 min	Existing dysfunctional habits should be replaced by new and helpful ones	Identified "thieves of time" from the mind-map (week 1) should be regarded more in detail
Organizing the flood of e-mails	About 25 min/week	Promotion of structured procedure	Long-term Organizing of e-mails, presenting methods
Written planning of my time	30 min/week	Encouragement for planning of short-term, middle-term and long-term activities	Stressing advantages of written planning,
The goal-means-analysis	25 min	Attempting aims structured and effectivly, promoting motivation	Learning the planning of goals through specific sub-steps
Serenity			
Who needs brooding?	–	Finding personal and individually effective signal for dysfunctional thoughts	Informing about the disadvantages through brooding, learning about the tool "signal"

with them. This made it clear for the participants how much they had achieved and experienced in the past 3 weeks.

Which Specific Contents Did the Training Have?

In the following two exercises are explained exemplarily. Further information can be found in Table 5.13. The basis of most of the exercises was next to the solution- and resources-oriented way of working primarily the work of Frank (2010), Lyubomirsky (2008), Seligman (2004) and Seiwert (2014). There is also overlap with the work of Ankenbrand and Gräfe (see Chaps. 5.1 and 5.2).

Serenity.

Example: *Your daily troublemakers*

To raise motivation the participants received a short overview about the advantages of patience. Aspects such as "health problems like headaches result from lacking patience" should give an additional reason to deal with the topic *serenity*. Contents were developed that deal with the detailed description of the current state in terms of "Which situations in your daily life get yourself worked up?". Afterwards followed a visualization of the successful future: "Assuming that you were able to react calmly, how could that work? How would you or others notice?". It is assumed that this state had already been reached at least partially, therefore it is taken up and explored how this situation was as well as how it was coped with. Finally the insights should be transferred to future situations: "How can you use your newly gained knowledge to find a way to react calmly in future, similar situations?".

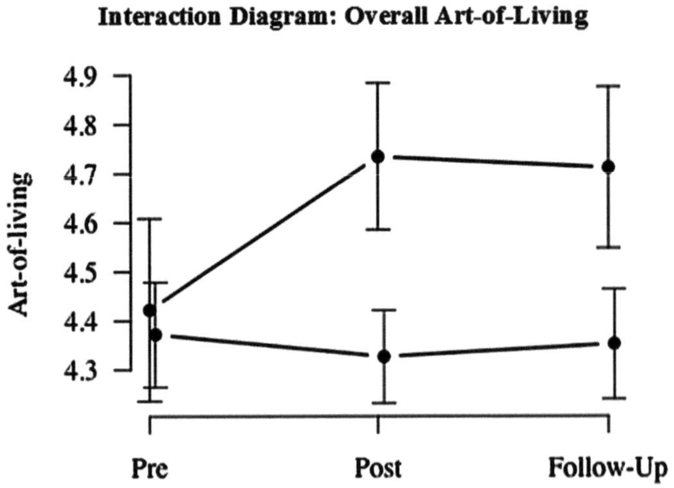

Fig. 5.17 Changes in *overall art-of-living* over the three times of measurement

Self-efficacy.

Example: *Your personal life-line*

The original exercise stems from Frank (2010) and deals with the life-line up to now. Ups and downs are marked and labeled on a number line. The emphasis should be on positive events and times in life. This also implies adverse circumstances that were coped with and overcome. Additionally value should be attached to resources. This means that the resulting life line should be examined more closely with positive and resources-oriented questions ("What did I manage well so far? How did I overcome downs or difficult times? Which strengths and resources helped me with this? In what way have I developed through my experiences? Resulting strengths?"). This exercise should also benefit the participants that have difficulties naming positive aspects or strengths deliberately.

5.4.4 Results

5.4.4.1 Quantitative Results

Firstly a repeated-measures analysis of variance with the within factors time (pretest, posttest, follow-up) and the between factor group (EG, CG) was conducted. The dependent variables were the *satisfaction with life scale* (SWLS) as well as the *art-of-living* overall value of the short version.

The analyses of variance showed significant interactions between time and group for the *art-of-living overall* value with $F(2, 84) = 8.28$, $p < .001$, $\eta^2 = .15$ as well as for satisfaction with life $F(2, 84) = 8.68$, $p < .001$, $\eta^2 = .17$. To test the effectiveness of the training for these variables, dependent t tests were conducted. Significant increases in the art-of-living overall means in the experimental group

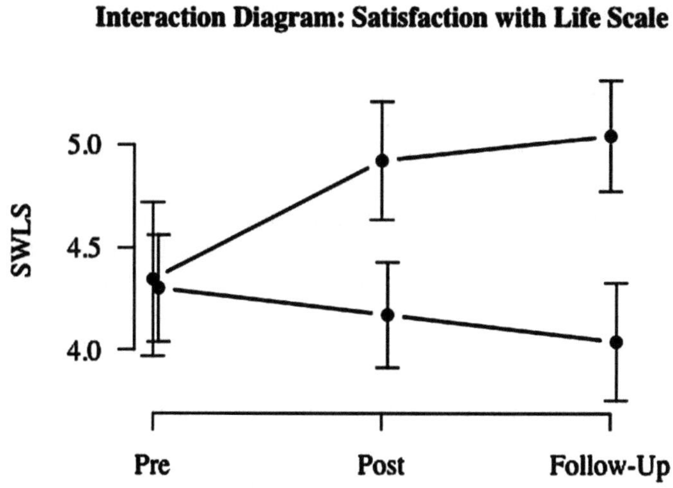

Fig. 5.18 Changes in *satisfaction with life* over the three times of measurement

were found between pre- to post-test with $t(25) = 4.60$, $p < .001$, $d = .47$ (see Fig. 5.17). For the SWLS changes with a medium effect size could also be shown, $t(25) = 3.33$, $p < .005$, $d = .41$ (see Fig. 5.18). The corresponding values of the control group remained stable over all three times of measurement. Comparisons between the second and the third time of measurement could display the stability of the training effect over 4 weeks for the *art-of-living overall* mean did not show significant changes from posttest to follow-up.

5.4.4.2 Qualitative Evaluation of the Training

The analyses of the evaluation questions (for N = 26) during the posttest or the follow-up showed that the exercises are includable in the every-day life to 81 % and were described as "exciting" and "versatile". Moreover the training was described as "helpful" (71 %) and it was said that it lead to a positive improvement (77 %). The participants could further choose single sub-components of the training which had improved in their opinion. Subjective improvements were reached for *serenity* (62 %), *physical care* (42 %), *optimization* (54 %) as well as for *self-efficacy* (35 %).

For a detailed evaluation, the participants could furthermore rate the individual exercises on a scale from *No, absolutely not helpful* to *Yes, absolutely helpful*. The results showed that the exercises *life-line* (77 %), *daily troublemakers* (81 %), the second unit about *physical health and fitness in the every-day life* (77 %), the *well-being diary* (77 %), the *radical acceptance* (69 %) and the voluntary exercise about *saying no* (72 %) were perceived as the most helpful ones. Overall, the combination of videos and written instructions as well as the preparation of expert knowledge in a comprehensible way was especially appreciated.

5.4.5 *Discussion*

5.4.5.1 Effectiveness of the Online-Training

The effectiveness for both the overall art-of-living scale and SWLS could be confirmed for the 3-week duration of the intervention as well as for the 4-week follow-up period. The training at hand could show like previous ones by Manthey et al. (2014) and Murray et al. (2015) that a purely online intervention without direct contact to the instructor is effective. Already studied techniques were deliberately used for this web-based training, which were as a consequence a good basis for the intervention. The concept of videos, combined with written instructions to download and the design of the training over 3 weeks seem to have been an effective combination, too. To focus on letting the participants find out for themselves what is already going good and what is improvable trains them to identify their own resources (e.g. perseverance), needs and goals.

5.4.5.2 Limitations

Finally only a small sample size could be implemented. A critical factor could here be the scheduled period of time which was during the holidays and thus during a potential vacation. Moreover, there was a number of dropouts. Besides, only a follow-up period of 4 weeks could be realized in this context, but to show a really stable effect of the training a longer period of time for the follow-up should be chosen in future studies. In addition to the short follow-up period, the duration of the training should be further enhanced.

A great number of participants stated that they needed more time and suggested a period of 5–6 weeks. At the same time, some of the participants found it difficult to invent the time needed for training participation. Especially for the first week (week of identification) more time would have been necessary. An even more individual support was wished for, since the maintaining of motivation in the everyday life was experienced as difficult.

5.4.5.3 Conclusion

Overall, the identified changes allow the conclusion that the exercises about art-of-living had their intended effect and that both art-of-living and well-being (SWLS) could be improved through the intervention. Furthermore, the interactions with medium effect sizes for these scales show stable values over the 4-week long follow-up period. This type of web-based training thus proved to be promising.

References

Bannink, F. P. (2012). *Praxis der positiven Psychologie* [The praxis of positive psychology]. Göttingen: Hogrefe Verlag.

Bao, K. J., & Lyubomirsky, S. (2014). Making happiness last: Using the hedonic adaptation prevention model to extend the success of positive interventions. In Parks, A. (Ed.), *The Wiley-Blackwell handbook of positive psychological inventions* (pp. 373–384). New York: Wiley-Interscience.

Baumgardner, S. R., & Crothers, M. K. (2010). *Positive psychology*. New Jersey: Pearson.

Beck, R., & Rush, J. S. B. F., & Emery, G. (1979). *Cognitive therapy of depression*. New York: Guilford press.

Beck, A. T., Steer, R. A., & Brown, G. K. (1996). *Beck Depression Inventory—Second edition: Manual*. San Antonio, TX: The Psychological Corporation.

Beitel, E. (1999). *Bochumer Gesundheitstraining. Ein ganzheitliches Übungsprogramm.* [An holistic training program]. Dortmund: Verlag modernes lernen.

Berg, J. M., Dutton, J. E., & Wrzesniewski, A. (2013). Job crafting and meaningful work. In B. J. Dik, Z. S. Byrne, & M. F. Steger (Eds.), *Purpose and meaning in the workplace* (pp. 81–104). Washington, DC: American Psychological Association.

Berking, M. (2008). *Training emotionaler Kompetenzen* [Trainng of emotional competences]. Heidelberg: Medizin Springer.

Besser, R. (2004). *Transfer: Damit Seminare Früchte tragen. Strategien, Übungen und Methoden, die eine konkrete Umsetzung in die Praxis sichern* [Transfer: Making seminars bear fruit. Strategies, exercises and methods to ensure practical implementation]. Weinheim, Basel: Beltz.

Blumenthal, J. A., Babyak, M. A., Moore, K. A., Craighead, E., Herman, S., Khatri, M., et al. (1999). Effects of exercise training on older patients with major depression. *Archives of Internal Medicine, 159*, 2349–2356.

Bolier, L., Haverman, M., Westerhof, G. J., Riper, H., Smit, F., & Bohlmeijer, E. (2013). Positive psychology interventions: a meta-analysis of randomized controlled studies. *BMC public health, 13*(1), 1. doi:10.1186/1471-2458-13-119.

Brock, R. L., Barry, R. A., Lawrence, E., Dey, J., & Rolffs, J. (2012). Internet administration of paper-and-pencil questionnaires used in couple research: Assessing psychometric equivalence. *Assessment, 19*, 226–242.

Buckingham, M., & Clifton, D. O. (2001). *Now, discover your strengths*. New York: Simon and Schuster.

Cohen, J. (1988). *Statistical power analysis for the behavioral sciences* (2nd ed.). Hillsdale: Lawrence Erlbaum Associates.

Cohn, M. A., & Fredrickson, B. L. (2010). In search of durable positive psychology interventions: Predictors and consequences of long-term positive behavior change. *The Journal of Positive Psychology, 5*, 355–366.

Cole, S. M., Bedeian, A. G., & Feild, H. S. (2006). The measurement equivalence of web- based and paper-and-pencil measures of transformational leadership. *Organizational Research Methods, 9*, 339–368.

Danner, D. D., Snowdon, D. A., & Friesen, W. V. (2001). Positive emotions in early life and longevity: Findings from the nun study. *Journal of Personality and Social Psychology, 80*, 804–813.

Diegelmann, C. (2007). *Trauma und Krise bewältigen* [Overcoming trauma and crisis]. Stuttgart: Klett-Cotta.

Diener, E. (1984). Subjective well-being. *Psychological Bulletin, 59*(3), 542–575.

Diener, E., Emmons, R. A., Larsen, R. J., & Griffin, S. (1985). The satisfaction with life scale. *Journal of Personality Assessment, 49*, 71–75.

Diener, E., & Lucas, R. (1999). Personality and subjective well-being. In D. Kahneman, E. Diener, & N. Schwarz (Eds.), *Well-being: The foundations of hedonic psychology* (pp. 213–229). New York: Sage.

D'Zurilla, T. J., & Goldfried, M. R. (1971). Problem solving and behavior modification. *Journal of Abnormal Psychology, 78*(1), 107–126.

Ellis, A. (1994). *Reason and emotion in psychotherapy. A comprehensive method of treating human disturbances. Revised and updated*. New York: Birch Lane Press.

Emmons, R. A., & McCullough, M. E. (2003). Counting blessings versus burdens: An experimental investigation of gratitude and subjective well-being in daily life. *Journal of Personality and Social Psychology, 84*, 277–289.

Fellmann, F. (2009). *Philosophie der Lebenskunst zur Einführung* [The philosophy of art-of-living for beginners]. Hamburg: Junius.

Foersterling, F. (1985). Attributional retraining: A review. *Psychological Bulletin, 98*, 495–512.

Fordyce, M. W. (1977). Development of a program to increase personal happiness. *Journal of Counseling Psychology, 24*, 511–521.

Frank, R. (2010). *Wohlbefinden fördern – Positive Therapie in der Praxis* [Enhancing well-being – The praxis of positive therapy]. Stuttgart: Klett-Cotta.

Fredrickson, B. L. (1998). What good are positive emotions? *Review of General Psychology, 2*, 300–319.

Fredrickson, B. L. (2001). The role of positive emotions in positive psychology: The broaden-and-build theory of positive emotion. *American Psychologist, 56*, 218–226.

Fredrickson, B. L. (2011). *Die Macht der guten Gefühle: Wie eine positive Haltung ihr Leben dauerhaft verändert* [The power of positive emotions: How a positve attitude can change your life]. Frankfurt am Main: Campus Verlag.

Fredrickson, B. L., Tugade, M. M., Waugh, C. E., & Larkin, G. (2003). What good are positive emotions in crises? A prospective study of resilience and emotions following the terrorist attacks on the United States on September 11th, 2001. *Journal of Personality and Social Psychology, 84*, 365–376.

Gander, F., René, T. P., Ruch, W., & Wyss, T. (2012). Strength-based positive interventions: Further evidence for their potential in enhancing well-being. *Journal of Happiness Studies*. doi:10.1007/s10902-012-9380-0.

Gilman, R., Huebner, E. S., & Furlong, M. J. (2009). *Handbook of positive psychology in schools*. New York, London: Routledge.

Glaesmer, H., Grande, G., Braehler, E., & Roth, M. (2011). The German Version of the Satisfaction with Life Scale—Psychometric Properties and Population based norms. *European Journal of Psychological Assessment, 27*, 127–132.

Glaesmer, H., Hoyer, J., Klotsche, J., & Herzberg, P. Y. (2008). Die deutsche Version des Life-Orientation-Tests (LOT-R) zum dispositionellen Optimismus und Pessimismus. [The German version of the Life-Orientation-Test (LOT-R) for measuring dispositional optimism and pessimism]. *Zeitschrift für Gesundheitspsychologie, 16*, 26–31.

Grant, A. M. (2007). Relational job design and the motivation to make a prosocial difference. *Academy of Management Review, 32*(2), 393–417.

Hackman, J. R., & Oldham, G. R. (1980). *Work redesign*. Reading, MA: Addison-Wesley.

Hanh, T. N. (1988). *The sun my heart: From mindfulness to insight contemplation*. California: Parallax Happiness Studies.

Hautzinger, M., Keller, F., & Kühner, C. (2009). *BDI-II. Beck-Depressions-Inventar. Revision* (2. Aufl.) [Revision of the BDI-II (2nd ed.)]. Frankfurt: Pearson Assessment.

Hone, L. C., Jarden, A., Schofield, G. M., & Duncan, S. (2014). Measuring flourishing: The impact of operational definitions on the prevalence of high levels of wellbeing. *International Journal of Wellbeing, 4*(1), 62–90. doi:10.5502/ijw.v4i1.4.

Inglehart, R., Foa, R., Peterson, C., & Welzel, C. (2008). Development, freedom, and rising happiness: A global perspective, 1981-2007. *Perspectives on Psychological Science, 3*, 264–285.

Jacobson, E. (2011). *Entspannung als Therapie: Progressive Relaxation in Therapie und Praxis*. [You must relax]. Stuttgart: Klett-Cotta

Kabat-Zinn, J., & Hanh, T. N. (2009). *Full catastrophe living: Using the wisdom of your body and mind to face stress, pain, and illness*. New York: Delta.

Kaluza, G. (2005). Stressbewältigung: Trainingsmanual zur psychologischen Gesundheitsförderung [Managing stress: Training manual for psychological health promotion]. Heidelberg: Springer.

King, L. A. (2001). The health benefits of writing about life goals. *Personality and Social Psychology Bulletin, 27*, 798–807.

Klauer, K. J., & Leutner, D. (2007). *Lehren und Lernen. Einführung in die Instruktionspsychologie* [Teaching and learning: An introduction to instructional psychology]. Weinheim: Beltz Psychologie Verlags Union.

Korotitsch, W., & Nelson Gray, R. O. (1999). An overview of self-monitoring research in assessment. *Psychological Assessment, 11*(4), 415–425.

Lammers, C. H. (2011). *Emotionsbezogene Psychotherapie: Grundlagen, Strategien und Techniken*. Stuttgart: Schattauer.

Landmann, M., & Schmitz, B. (Hrsg.). (2007). *Selbstregulation erfolgreich fördern. Praxisnahe Trainingsprogramme für effektives Lernen* [Facitating self-regulated learning: practical training-programs to ensure effective learning]. Stuttgart: Kohlhammer.

Lopez, S. J., Pedrotti, J. T., & Snyder, C. R. (2014). *Positive psychology—The scientific and practical explorations of human strengths*. London: Sage.

Lyubomirsky, S. (2008). *The how of happiness: A scientific approach to getting the life you want*. New York: Penguin Press.

Lyubomirsky, S., King, L., & Diener, E. (2005a). The benefits of frequent positive affect: Does happiness lead to success? *Psychological Bulletin, 131*, 803–855.

Lyubomirsky, S., & Lepper, H. S. (1999). A measure of subjective happiness: Preliminary reliability and construct validation. *Social Indicators Research, 46*, 137–155.

Lyubomirsky, S., Sheldon, K. M., & Schkade, D. (2005b). Pursuing happiness: The architecture of sustainable change. *Review of General Psychology, 9*, 111–131.

Manthey, L., Vehreschild, V., & Renner, K. H. (2014). Effectiveness of two cognitive. Interventions promoting happiness with video-based online instructions. *Journal of Happiness Studies, 17*(1), 319–339.

Maruta, T., Colligan, R., Malinchoc, M., & Offord, K. (2000). Optimists vs. pessimists: Survival rate among medical patients over a 30-year period. *May Clinic Proceedings, 75*, 140–143.

Meier, R. (2005). *30 Minuten für mehr Glück und Zufriedenheit.* [30 minutes to enhance luck and satisfaction]. Offenbach: Gabal.

Murray, G., Leitan, N. D., Berk, M., Thomas, N., Michalak, E., Berk, L., et al. (2015). Online mindfulness-based intervention for late-stage bipolar disorder: Pilot evidence for feasibility and effectiveness. *Journal of Affective Disorders, 178*, 46–51.

Nürnberger, E (2010). *Optimistisch denken* [Thinking optimistically]. Freiburg: Haufe-Lexware.

Osgood, C. E. (1964). Semantic differential technique in the comparative study of cultures. *American Anthropologist, 66*, 171–200. doi:10.2307/669329.

Perels, F., van de Loo, K., & Schmitz, B. (2008). *Trainer trainieren: Seminare effektiv gestalten* [Teaching teachers: Make your seminars more effective]. Stuttgart: Kohlhammer.

Peterson, C., Park, N., & Seligman, M. E. P. (2005). Orientations to happiness and life satisfaction: The full versus the empty life. *Journal of Happiness Studies, 6*, 25–41.

Peterson, C., & Seligman, M. (2004). *Character strengths and virtues: A handbook and classification.* Oxford: Oxford University Press.

Pfennig, T. (2009). Die Macht der Selbsthypnose. [The power self-hypnosis]. Schrobenhausen: Rainer Bloch.

Reil, K. (2012). *Die Selbstreflexion der Studierenden fordern und fördern.* [Demanding and promotion self-reflection of students]. In R. Arntz, H. P. Krings & B. Kühn (Hrsg.,). Autonomie und Assessment - Erträge des 3. Bremer Symposions zum autonomen Fremdsprachenlernen (S. 204–208). Bochum: AKS.

Roth, G. (2007). Persönlichkeit, Entscheidung und Verhalten: Warum es so schwierig ist, sich und andere zu ändern. [Personality, decisions and behaviour: Why it is so difficult to change oneself and others]. Stuttgart: Klett-Cotta.

Ryan, R. M., & Deci, E. L. (2000). Self-determination theory and the facilitation of intrinsic motivation, social development, and well-being. *American Psychologist, 55*(1), 68.

Scheier, M. F., Carver, C. S., & Bridges, M. W. (1994). Distinguishing optimism from neuroticism (and trait anxiety, self-mastery, and self-esteem): A re-evaluation of the Life Orientation Test. *Journal of Personality and Social Psychology, 67*, 1063–1078.

Schmid, W. (1998). *Philosophie der Lebenskunst. Eine Grundlegung* [The philosophy of art-of-living]. Frankfurt am Main: Suhrkamp.

Schmid, W. (2007). *Mit sich selbst befreundet sein: Von der Lebenskunst im Umgang mit sich selbst.* [To be freinds with ourselves] Frankfurt a. M.: Suhrkamp.

Schmitz, B., & Perels, F. (2011). Self-monitoring of self-regulation during math homework behaviour using standardized diaries. *Metacognition and Learning, 6*(3), 255–273.

Schmitz, B., & Schmidt, A. (2014). Entwicklung eines Fragebogens zur Lebenskunst. *Pychologie in Erziehung und Unterricht, 61*(4), 252–266.

Schmitz, B., & Wiese, B. (2006). New perspectives for the evaluation of training sessions in self-regulated learning: Time series-analyses of diary data. *Contemporary Educational Psychology, 31*, 64–96.

Schueller, S. M., & Seligman, M. E. P. (2010). Pursuit of pleasure, engagement, and meaning: Relationships to subjective and objective measures of well-being. *The Journal of Positive Psychology, 5*, 253–263.

Schwarz, N., & Strack, F. (1999). Reports of subjective well-being: Judgmental processes and their methodological implications. In D. Kahneman, E. Diener & N. Schwarz (Eds.), *Well-being: The foundation of hedonic psychology* (pp. 61–84). New York: Sage.

Schwarzer, R., & Jerusalem, M. (2002). Das Konzept der Selbstwirksamkeit [The concept of self-efficacy]. *Zeitschrift für Pädagogik, 44*, 28–53.

Seiffge-Krenke, I. (2006). *Nach PISA. Stress in der Schule und mit den Eltern* [After PISA. The struggle with school and parents.]. *Bewältigungskompetenz deutscher Jugendlicher im internationalen Vergleich.* Göttingen: Vandenhoeck & Ruprecht.

Seiwert, L.J. (1995). *Das neue 1x1 des Zeitmanagement* [Modern time management 101]. Offenbach: Gabal.

Seiwert, L. (2014). *Das 1 x 1 des Zeitmanagement: Zeiteinteilung, Selbstbestimmung, Lebensbalance* [The basics of time management: time-allocation, self-determination and work-life-balance]. München: Gräfe und Unzer. 2. Auflage.

Seligman, M. E. (2004). *Authentic happiness: Using the new positive psychology to realize your potential for lasting fulfillment*. Simon and Schuster.

Seligman, M. E. (2011). *Learned optimism: How to change your mind and your life*. Vintage.

Seligman, M. E. (2012). *Flourish: A visionary new understanding of happiness and well-being*. New York: Simon and Schuster.

Seligman, M. E. P., & Csikszentmihalyi, M. (2000). Positive psychology: An introduction. *American Psychologist, 55*, 5–14.

Seligman, M. E., Ernst, R. M., Gillham, J., Reivich, K., & Linkins, M. (2009). Positive education: Positive psychology and classroom interventions. *Oxford Review of Education, 35*(3), 293–311.

Seligman, M. E. P., Steen, T. A., Park, N., & Peterson, C. (2005). Positive psychology progress: Empirical validation of interventions. *American Psychologist, 60*, 410–421.

Sheldon, K. M., & Lyubomirsky, S. (2006). How to increase and sustain positive emotion: The effects of expressing gratitude and visualizing best possible selves. *The Journal of Positive Psychology, 1*, 73–82.

Silberman, M. L. (1990). *Active training*. New York: Lexington books.

Sin, N. L., & Lyubomirsky, S. (2009). Enhancing well-being and alleviating depressive symptoms with positive psychology interventions: A practice-friendly meta-analysis. *Journal of Clinical Psychology, 65*, 467–487. doi:10.1002/jclp.20593.

Steger, M. F., & Dik, B. J. (2009). work as meaning: Individual and organizational benefits of engaging in meaningful work. In P. A. Linley, S. Harrington & N. Garcea (Eds.), *Oxford handbook of positive psychology and work* (pp. 131–141). New York: Oxford University Press.

Stepper, S., & Strack, F. (1993). Proprioceptive determinants of emotional and nonemotional feelings. *Journal of Personality and Social Psychology, 64*, 211–220.

Strack, F., Martin, L., & Stepper, S. (1988). Inhibiting and facilitating conditions of the human smile: A nonobtrusive test of the facial feedback hypothesis. *Journal of Personality and Social Psychology, 54*, 768–777.

Tabachnick, B. G., & Fidell, L. S. (2013). *Using multivariate statistics* (6th ed.). Boston: Pearson Education.

Tugade, M. M., & Fredrickson, B. L. (2004). Resilient individuals use positive emotions to bounce back from negative emotional experiences. *Journal of Personality and Soial Psychology, 86*, 320–333.

University of Leicester. (2006). Psychologist produces the first-ever 'World Map Of Happiness'. *Science Daily*. Retrieved 02 Sep 2016 from http://www.sciencedaily.com/releases/2006/11/061113093726.htm.

Veenhoven, R. (2003a). Arts-of-living. *Journal of Happiness Studies, 4*, 373–384.

Veenhoven, R. (2003b). Notions of art-of-living. *Journal of Happness Studies, 4*, 345–349.

Wagnild, G., & Young, H. (1993). Development and psychometric. *Journal of Nursing Measurement, 1*(2), 165–178.

Wengenroth, M. (2012). *Therapie-Tools Akzeptanz- und Commitmenttherapie (ACT)* [Therapy-tools: acceptance- and commitment-therapy (ACT)]. Weinheim: Beltz.

World Health Organization. (1948). World health organization constitution. *Basic documents, 1*. Retrieved 02 Sep 2016 from http://www.who.int/governance/eb/who_constitution_en.pdf.

Wrzesniewski, A., McCauley, C. R., Rozin, P., & Schwartz, B. (1997). Jobs, careers, and callings: People's relations to their work. *Journal of Research in Personality, 31*(1), 21–33.

Chapter 6
Summary and Outlook

6.1 Art-of-Living in the Arts

Sarah Haardt, Jana Demel, Janina Linten and Thomas Proksch

In this section we present examples of art-of-living strategies which can be found in the arts. Art-of-living strategies are widely spread over all art forms and can be found in movies, theater plays, novels and autobiographies. Due to the extensiveness of this research field it is not within the limits of this book to give a complete review of representations of art-of-living in the arts. We rather want to give some impressions on how art-of-living can be found in everyday life.

If one is interested in the occurrence of positive psychology in movies there already exists an interesting series of books by Niemic and Wedding (2008, 2014), although the authors, differently from our approach, are associated with the tradition of strength and virtues (cf. Chap. 2, 3). They also have a higher aspiration level regarding the effects of these movies as they express that "Most of the 24 strengths can be potentially elicited in the viewer as direct result of the film" (Niemiec and Wedding 2008, p. 8).

Within the scope of this book we focus on autobiographies as they allow the analysis of the original phrasing of the authors and need not be interpreted too much. We arbitrarily chose five famous persons to reflect on as well as five sub-components corresponding to that persons' life. It would have been easy to find more examples but we did not expect high additional effects from that.

The famous individuals are to be found in different areas of life: Luciano Pavarotti, a singer of classical opera, the Dalai Lama, a religious leader, Henry Thoreau, a writer, Eric Clapton, a pop-music interpreter, and Nelson Mandela, a political leader. The exemplified subcomponents are *savoring*, *openness*, *serenity*, *coping* and *self-determined way of living*. Our approach is the following: For each

B. Schmitz, *Art-of-Living*, Social Indicators Research Series 63,
DOI 10.1007/978-3-319-45324-8_6

Table 6.1 Author of the autobiography, title of the publication and art-of-living strategy which is exemplified

Autobiographer	Title	Strategy
Luciano Pavarotti	My World	Savoring
Dalai Lama	My Spiritual Autobiography	Openness
Eric Clapton	Eric Clapton: the autobiography	Coping
Henry David Thoreau	Walden	Serenity
Nelson Mandela	Long Walk To Freedom	Self-determined manner of living

subcomponent we shortly refer to its meaning within art-of-living, then we give very short information on the biography of the person and finally we present information how the famous person is related to the art-of-living subcomponent.

Table 6.1 gives an overview of authors and strategies.

6.1.1 Savoring/Pavarotti

The medium through which savoring is practiced is of little importance: Music, food, wellness as well as physical activities or art can all be the source of a pleasant experience. Its quality, however, is defined by the individual's attentiveness to it. Yet savoring is a strategy allowing for remarkable individual differences, as the aforementioned experiences can only be interpreted from a person's subjective point of view.

A remarkable representative for savoring as an art-of-living strategy can be found in the world-famous singer Luciano Pavarotti. Not only did his physical appearance seem to portray him as a symbol of savoring, but he also managed to integrate savoring into nearly all domains of his stressful everyday life.

"I'm like a man who eats rich food and drinks good wine all year long." (Pavarotti and Wright 1998, p. 312). Born in Modena in 1935, Pavarotti rose to fame as one of the world's most influential tenors who did not limit himself to classical music and the opera, but also created duets with numerous pop-idols. He continued to utilize his fame and success to support the Red Cross and other humanitarian institutions with charity concerts until he died at the age of 71 in Modena.

However, he did not limit his savoring to exquisite food and wine but deliberately chose to go on downtime multiple times, retreating from the view of the public eye in order to spend time with his family. In doing so he emphasized the importance of relaxation under the absence of any pressure of time. Even during his worldwide tours Pavarotti seized numerous opportunities which he dedicated to nothing but savoring. He consciously experienced these moments, observing how they positively affected his emotional state. "Everyone has a good side and it is up to you to find that side. [If] you waste your time looking at the negative (…), you will always find plenty that is bad and never find the good side." (Pavarotti and Wright 1998, p. 262).

Pavarotti's savoring can be described as diverse which is probably best illustrated by his stance on women: He greatly appreciated their company and also noticed their positive effects on his well-being.

In summary, one has to recognize Luciano Pavarotti's ability of consciously perceiving and seizing the enjoyable opportunities life provides—his ability to savor the moment. Using this art-of-living strategy both enhanced his well-being and enabled him to manage his stressful daily routine.

6.1.2 Openness/Dalai Lama

Schmid (2004) believes openness to be a necessary requirement for art-of-living, describing it as critically approaching existing norms, being eager to handle them in an unconventional manner as well as deliberately striving to make new experiences.

We find Tenzin Gyatso, the fourteenth Dalai Lama, to be an extraordinary example for the art-of-living strategy openness. Born in Tibet in 1935 he was declared the next Dalai Lama at the age of two and thereby challenged with the tasks of facilitating harmony between the various religions, or rather, the whole of humanity, in order to enable every person, family and the community to live a full and happy life. Regarded by many as a symbol of peace, in his autobiography the Dalai Lama elaborates on dire, challenging conflicts humanity faces. Profoundly criticizing religiously motivated wars he emphasizes the fundamental values of compassion and love.

Although his religious faith remains unchanged, Gyatso approaches other religions openly and with a genuine interest for interconfessional communication. Thereby the Dalai Lama frequently undertakes pilgrimages. "As I was looking at Mary, I felt rising up within me a sincere admiration and authentic respect for Christianity (…). The Christian religion does, of course, have a different philosophy from my own, but the aid and concrete benefits it brings are undeniable." (The Dalai Lama 2011, p. 84). However, Tenzin Gyatso also analyzes his own religion—Buddhism—from a critical point of view, freely recognizing its limitations and desiring to overcome the inherent barriers.

> (…) I have wanted to go beyond the borders of my faith to clarify certain universal principles, with the aim of helping everyone find happiness. (The Dalai Lama 2011, p. 105)

Moreover, Gyatso has always shown a remarkable interest for western culture. "(…) I have been very impressed by Western society, (…) especially (…) its energy, (…) creativity and its hunger for knowledge." (The Dalai Lama 2011, p. 108). Although constantly under severe political pressure, he has, at many times, proven his ability to critically, yet openly approach and address norms and values as well as social and political issues while maintaining a tolerant and interested attitude towards the western political systems as well as towards technology. Generally speaking the Dalai Lama excellently embodies the strategy *openness*.

6.1.3 Coping/Eric Clapton

Coping is regarded as the strategy of managing and overcoming unpleasant and painful experiences, for example death or illness, with which an individual might be faced. It enables artists-of-living to acquire further strategies for overcoming blows of fate. Famous musician and 20-times Grammy-Award winner Eric Clapton suffered many severe crises in his life and still managed to return to a stable, happy and joyful state of mind. We will therefore illustrate *coping* referring to his exemplary experiences and life choices.

In 1945 he was born into a family often unavailable, which led Clapton to his ongoing love of music, on which he relied heavily in order to compensate his troubles at home."Music became a healer for me, and I learned to listen with all my being. I found that it could wipe away all the emotion of fear and confusion relating to my family." (Clapton and Sykes 2007, p. 16). "I found my God in music and the arts (…). (…) God was always there, but now I have learned to talk to him." (Clapton and Sykes 2007, pp. 257). This theme continued when Clapton struggled to overcome the tragic death of his beloved son Conor, which he mourns in his most famous song to date, "Tears in Heaven". "Originally, these songs were never meant for publication or public consumption, they were just what I did to stop from going mad." (Clapton and Sykes 2007, p. 274). The remarkable success of these expressive songs facilitated Clapton's fame, making him one of the most influential blues-rock musicians in the world.

Music, however, was not the only source of support Clapton could draw from: Having suffered from a severe alcohol and drug addiction he joined a twelve-step-sobriety-program, whose fellow members he still considers his friends. "Many people might have thought (…) that I would ultimately drink, but I had the fellowship, and I had my guitar." (Clapton and Sykes 2007, p. 272). In addition, Clapton could rely on colleagues and friends he had met during his years of touring the world, but also his own daughter Ruth. In 2002 he married his third wife, Melia McEnery, with whom he has three daughters. "[The letter was] (…) from Keith Richards; it just said: "If there is anything I can do, just let me know." I'll always be grateful for that." (Clapton and Sykes 2007, p. 268). "I realise what a profound effect (…)[Ruth] had on my well-being as a whole." (Clapton and Sykes 2007, p. 275).

Eric Clapton illustrates perfectly how drawing from resources can enable an artist-of-living to cope with even the direst situations and tragedies.

6.1.4 Serenity/Henry David Thoreau

An artist-of-living who makes use of the strategy *serenity* develops an attitude of acceptance and internalizes that it is not necessary to constantly control and influence the environment. Thus, radiating from such a person is a feeling of relaxation and calmness (Schmid 2004).

American writer and philosopher Henry David Thoreau decided to abandon his societal responsibilities and belongings in order to retreat to a life of utmost simplicity and solitude, free from social conventions and pressure of time. We therefore deem him to be an excellent symbol for the strategy *serenity*.

"While I enjoy the friendship of the seasons I trust that nothing can make life a burden to me." (Thoreau 2014, p. 73). After struggling with his profession as a teacher, because he refused to make use of corporal punishment which was deemed to be of vital importance at the time, he founded his own private school which closed its doors in 1842 after the death of Thoreau's brother. Retreating to the forests, he reduced his life to a minimum and aimed his endeavors at identifying what is truly essential in life. However, he did so without any schedule similar to those typical in society. "Every morning was a cheerful invitation to make my life of equal simplicity and (…) innocence, with nature itself. (…) It matters not what the clocks say or the attitudes and labors of men. Morning is when I am awake and there is a dawn in me." (Thoreau 2014, p. 50). Thoreau continues to emphasize the importance of living in the moment, discarding fear of the future or anticipation as well as melancholy and mourning of the past. "There were times when I could not afford to sacrifice the bloom of the present moment to any work, whether of the head or the hands." (Thoreau 2014, p. 62)

Living a serene life was his utmost priority. Constantly striving for success and improvement to him seemed unnecessary as it took up too much time and resources without producing outcomes truly essential for a full life. "We should not meet thus in haste." (Thoreau 2014, p. 91).

After his time in extreme remoteness, Thoreau returned to his home town, while maintaining his austere lifestyle. Until the day he succumbed to a bronchitis in 1962, he was an outspoken advocate for civil disobedience and continued to live a life of calm simplicity. Therefore, he could be viewed as person to illustrate the strategy *serenity*.

6.1.5 Self-Determined Way of Living/Mandela

Everyone has an intuitive grasp of the meaning behind the art-of-living strategy *self-determined way of living*: Acting according to one's individual values and norms while determining priorities oneself, regardless of the social environment's stance towards such behavior, results in a more profound feeling of meaning. This strategy is brilliantly portrayed by the first dark-skinned South-African president, an outspoken political activist and firm opposer of Apartheid, Nelson Mandela.

"Education is the great engine of personal development. It is through education that the daughter of a peasant can become a doctor, that the son of a mineworker can become head of the mine (…). It is what we make out of what we have, not what we are given, that separates one person from another." (Mandela 1995,

p. 166). This quote impressively summarizes the essence of Mandela's philosophy. Born in 1918 the young Mandela was sent to school, which was unusual at the time. In doing so however, his parents laid the cornerstone for his career early on.

> I felt many of my established beliefs (…) begin to ebb away. In that instant, I saw that life might hold more for me than being a champion stick-fighter. (Mandela 1995, p. 16)

After his father's death, the young Mandela became a regent's protégé, as a result of which his financial situation and status increased drastically. Even though he was thankful for the generosity, when the regent decided to arrange a marriage for Mandela, he fled to Johannesburg.

> I was a romantic and I was not prepared to have anyone, even the regent select a bride for me. (Mandela 1995, p. 54) (…) the only option remaining was to run away. (Mandela 1995, p. 55)

It was during his time in Johannesburg that Mandela advanced his political career, culminating in the better-known chapter of his life: After 27 years of incarceration as a result of his activities against Apartheid he was set free in 1990. Four years later, in 1994, he was democratically elected for president, which he should remain until 1999. When he died in Johannesburg in 2013, the world lost a firm advocate of humanitarian causes and race equality. His incredible persistence and his remarkable dedication to his values make him a good example for the strategy *self-determined way of living.*

6.1.6 Summary: Art-of-Living in the Arts

These examples are in no way exhaustive for art-of-living strategies in autobiographies nor have all art-of-living strategies been exemplified. The selection is rather arbitrary and serves only for demonstration purposes. We selected these authors because they are famous to a greater audience and therefore, most people need only short descriptions to understand which art-of-living strategy is exemplified by that person. We think that even only a few examples of famous people demonstrating strategies of art-of-living sub-components in their life may help to get a more vivid picture of how art-of-living could be found in real life.

6.2 Nomination Study for Art-of-Living

Alina Stöver, Monica Da Silva-Bettner and Alina Wuttke

In Sect. 6.1 we described famous people and interpreted aspects of their behavior with respect to at least one art-of-living sub-component. We did not present enough information on these people to decide whether they could be regarded as overall artists-of-living. One might get the impression that only very few people with extraordinary attitudes and behavior could be artists-of-living, but our approach assumes that most individuals could be artists-of-living and each individual could learn and enhance art-of-living strategies. Therefore, we now try to identify artists-of-living.

Do people know artists-of-living? How are artists-of-living characterized by other people? How do artists-of-living characterize themselves? Do they differ from normal people with respect to art-of-living? It can be assumed that people are able to learn art-of-living. To further understand what natural experts in the field of art-of-living find important and which strategies they really apply, it could prove useful to capture the whole range of resources, strategies and attitudes marking people that already successfully practice art-of-living.

Therefore the following study aimed to look at art-of-living in a broader sense and to learn directly from those who are living it (artists-of-living). For this purpose, people considered to be artists-of-living were found via nomination and interviewed as to get an impression which competences and approaches make them artists-of-living.

6.2.1 *Process of Nomination*

Before interviewing artists-of-living, the first step was to find them. To generate a sample we followed the method of Baltes et al. (1995) which was developed during the course of their wisdom research: They had asked experts, in their case journalists of different media in Berlin, to nominate "sages", restricted to public figures and politicians of Berlin to generate a high consensus. The study at hand was the first to use a nomination process in the area of art-of-living.

The original idea to nominate a sample comes from the Delphi-method (Häder 2002) which is useful in cases where the sought-after information does not originate from established knowledge. In this process, experts are asked to nominate people which fit certain criteria. The definition of an expert varies with the subject of the study and can, amongst others, include domain experts as well as affected persons. This is not only true for the experts but also for those who are nominated. A typical element of the Delphi-method is that the experts nominate a person matching the profile *anonymously*. Therefore, the study at hand used the method of a written, anonymized nomination based on the Delphi-method.

In the course of the study, a special "Rating method" was used to examine the importance and realization, meaning a practical, action-related realization, of the 17 areas of art-of-living for the artists-of-living. It included 17 cards with each having an art-of-living scale and a short description of the scale on the front and an example from the art-of-living questionnaire (cf. Chap. 2) on the back. During the course of the interview, the participants were supposed to assign the cards to different categories of importance and realization.

Also, the revised questionnaire of art-of-living (Chap. 2) was used as a basis for studying the expression of the 17 scales of art-of-living. The overall value for art-of-living consists of the overall values of the single scales. In the main study, its value for Cronbach's alpha was 0.92.

With these methods, quantitative data was generated. The following hypothesis was postulated:

H1: It is possible to identify artists of living. That means that the scores for art-of-living for the artists-of-living will be higher compared to the normal population, cf. Chap. 3.

As more explorative question we look at the importance and the realization the artists-of-living assign to the art-of-living sub-components. Which strategy do they find important, which one do they apply in their life? Do these ratings of importance and realization correspond to the results of the art-of-living questionnaire?

In addition to the quantitative approach, there was also a qualitative one, aiming to get an understanding of art-of-living from people who were already practicing it. This was investigated with open questions in interviews. With a content analysis of their answers, the corresponding principles or maxims were collected to find strategies and helpful attitudes towards life and to learn from them. This approach was explorative and therefore no hypotheses were formulated, but we will analyze whether their advice regarding strategies for art-of-living corresponds to the subscales of our questionnaire. We are also interested how artists-of-living view our concept measured by the questionnaire.

All in all, the investigation consisted of three studies: the pilot study, which served to test the instruments, the nomination study and the main study.

6.2.2 Nomination Study

The second study aimed to nominate and select artists-of-living. Two methods to get nominations took place, but the first one failed due to a very little response rate. Therefore, only the second approach and its results are described.

An online questionnaire was sent via e-mail to- and shared in social networks with friends of the investigators and fellow psychology students. It introduced the participants to the definition of art-of-living and asked whether they knew a person who was, in their opinion, actually living the concept. They were supposed to add additional information about this person such as name, e-mail-address, age and what makes it an artist-of-living. They could nominate up to seven people. Via the given e-mail-addresses, the potential subjects for the second study were contacted with a standardized e-mail containing information about the study in general and the procedure of the interview. Time and place for the interview were scheduled with people who answered within 2 weeks.

Overall, 49 people were nominated (including one person who was nominated twice), coming from all over Germany, and in the end, interviews with 40 of them could be arranged. 24 of the participants wrote short descriptions of the people they had nominated as artists-of-living. Aspects that were found very often were, e.g., an inspiring and exceptional life-style, a positive attitude and love of life and rising again after defeats und making the best of everything. To illustrate some facets of an artist-of-living, extracts will be presented.

> … inspires me with his life-style, the things that had priority in his life and his attitude towards life. I have experienced … as a very spiritual person who finds a balance between work and time for himself in silence. … is very modest and mindful.

> … is a artist-of-living to me, because she has got things straightened out with herself, when faced with difficulties, she keeps her chin up and approaches the issue with vigor and joy. She is mindful to herself by having a good contact with her body, feeling well and caring for herself. And she always brings me into a good mood, because she simply radiates a good feeling and security.

6.2.3 *Main Study*

In the main study, the nominated artists-of-living were interviewed. The interview consisted of two parts. The first one contained welcoming the participants and an introduction as well as open questions including two Rating methods. In the second part the participants filled in the art-of-living questionnaire.

6.2.3.1 Sample

All in all, 40 interviews were conducted of which two had to be eliminated due to methodological problems in the nomination process. The final sample (N = 38) consisted of 20 (52.6 %) women and 18 (47.4 %) men. Eight (21.1 %) participants reported to belong to the age group from 18 to 29, 13 (34.2 %) to the age group 30 to 45 and 17 (44.7 %) to be older than 45. 26 (68.4 %) participants were working, 12 (31.6 %) were not. 12 (31.6 %) people lived in a household with children under 18, whereas 26 did not (68.4 %).

All of the participants voluntarily took part in the study and signed an informed consent.

6.2.3.2 Interview Guideline

As one method of the study, a standardized interview conducted face to face was chosen (Atteslander 2010). Although interviews have methodological problems such as response bias, acquiescence bias or social desirability (Atteslander 2010), the method was chosen due to a critical advantage: the participants could open up in a familiar atmosphere and talk about their attitudes and personal experiences. The interview was conducted on the basis of a standardized questionnaire which qualified it as a strongly structured interview situation according to Schnell and Hill

(2013). For all participants "the same questions with the same formulation and order" were used (Schnell and Hill 2013, p. 315).

Each session was designed to last 90 min. Sixty minutes were planned for the interview including the Rating method, 30 min for answering the art-of-living questionnaire. The interview was conducted according to the interview guideline and consisted of seven steps which will be described in the following. Between step 6 and 7, the art-of-living questionnaire was integrated.

Step 1: Introduction

At first, the background of the study as well as the procedure was explained. Then the participants received information about the privacy policy and the voluntary nature of the participation and had the possibility to ask questions.

Step 2: Introduction to the topic

The first question was: "First of all we are interested briefly which experiences you already have with the topic art-of-living. What do you understand by art-of-living? What does art-of-living mean to you?"

Step 3: Comprehension

In the third step, background information about art-of-living was given to the participants to establish a basis for the further interview. Art-of-living was defined as conscious way of living and the 17 areas of art-of-living were introduced. It was also explained that the study assumed that every person considers the single areas as differently relevant in his own life. Subsequently the 17 cards with the art-of-living areas were given to the participants.

Step 4: Rating method

Next, the Rating method was conducted. The participants were asked to assign the cards to different categories according to the importance and realization.
The three categories of importance were:

- Rather very important in my current situation in life.
- Moderately important in my current situation in life.
- Less important in my current situation in life.

The three categories for the assessment of realization were:

- In my current situation in life I strongly live out this area.
- In my current situation in life I moderately live out this area.
- In my current situation in life I live out this area less strongly.

Step 5. Learning from artists-of-living

Two questions concretely asked for three principles in life or three values which direct one's actions as well as for strategies to stay true to these principles. Additionally, their attitudes and abilities or strategies that helped them to gain satisfaction with life were identified. This was done with an imagination task.

> Imagine you are standing before the cradle of a newborn. You have the special task to provide it with a little miracle bag. In this bag there are several ingredients which help the child to reach satisfaction with life. From your own personal experience, which ingredients

do you put into the little miracle bag? Which attitudes and abilities that help yourself do you want to give the child to take with him or her?

Step 6. Atmospheric picture (optional)
Step 7. Motto in life

In the last step, the participants were asked to spontaneously tell their personal motto in life.

6.2.4 *Results*

6.2.4.1 Data Analysis

The data from the questionnaire and the rating method was analyzed quantitatively whereby individual scales with more than 30 % missing values were eliminated.

The answers collected with the imagination task, asking for attitudes and abilities/strategies that helped the participants to gain satisfaction with life, were analyzed qualitatively with a content analysis. The data from further questions was used exemplarily.

6.2.4.2 Quantitative Analysis

Numeric values were assigned to the three levels of importance and realization whereby for both variables a high value was assigned the number three, a moderate value the number two and a low value was assigned the number one.

Results for Hypothesis 1

With our method of nomination we were able to identify artists-of-living which differed with high statistical significance from our normal population, cf. Table 6.2 as the overall score for art-of-living was significantly higher for artists of living than for the normal population. The greatest differences were found for *meaning*, *openness*, and *positive attitudes towards life* whereas the group means did not differ significantly for *integrating different areas of living*, *shaping of living conditions*, *reflection* and *savoring*.

Results for the Research Question

But what sub-constructs were given the most importance by the artists-of-living? Referring to the ranked order for the sub-constructs, we see in Table 6.3 that the most important were *social contact*, *positive attitude towards life*, *openness*, *self-*

Table 6.2 Differences between means scores for art-of-living and normal sample means, SD, N

Art-of-living scale	Normal sample			Artists-of-living			T-value for difference
	M	*SD*	*N*	*M*	*SD*	*N*	*t* (37)
Balance	4.53	0.73	636	4.86	0.53	38	3.64
Coping	3.80	0.70	636	4.22	0.63	38	3.97
Serenity	3.50	0.96	636	4.07	0.80	38	4.21
Savoring	4.41	0.72	636	4.55	0.70	38	1.20
Physical care	4.23	0.86	636	4.66	0.76	38	3.36
Integrating different areas of life	4.16	0.67	636	4.26	0.76	38	0.79
Openness	4.37	0.72	636	4.98	0.56	38	6.41
Optimization	4.19	0.57	636	4.58	0.50	38	4.63
Positive attitude towards life	4.57	0.75	636	5.07	0.52	38	5.59
Self-determined way of living	4.44	0.63	636	4.82	0.50	38	4.48
Social contact	4.80	0.68	636	5.02	0.55	38	2.36
Self-efficacy	4.16	0.66	636	4.62	0.61	38	4.49
Self-knowledge	4.56	0.66	636	4.86	0.49	38	3.58
Shaping of living conditions	4.80	0.70	636	4.92	0.66	38	1.08
Self-actualization	4.73	0.62	636	5.10	0.55	38	4.00
Reflection	4.67	0.66	636	4.62	0.53	38	0.56
Meaning	4.66	0.72	636	5.25	0.43	38	7.83
Overall Art-of-living score	4.39	0.35	636	4.73	0.33	38	6.15

Table 6.3 Means and ranks for ratings of the artists-of-living for realization and importance of their art-of-living strategies

Art-of-living strategies	Realization		Importance	
	M	*Rank*	*M*	*Rank*
Balance	2.00	12	2.05	11
Optimization	1.89	15	1.76	17
Self-determined way of living	2.42	5	2.24	6
Self-knowledge	2.14	8	1.97	13
Physical care	2.05	10	2.18	7
Savoring	1.82	16	2.08	10
Coping	2.11	9	1.95	14.5
Positive attitude towards life	2.58	1	2.49	2
Serenity	2.00	12	2.16	8
Openness	2.45	3.5	2.42	3
Social contact	2.24	7	2.53	1
Shaping of living conditions	1.95	14	1.81	16
Integrating different areas of living	1.71	17	1.95	14.5
Self-actualization	2.00	12	2.00	12
Reflection	2.32	6	2.32	5
Meaning	2.45	3.5	2.11	9
Self-efficacy	2.47	2	2.41	4

efficacy, *reflection* and *self-determined way of living*. The Spearman rank order correlations between art-of-living and importance turned out to be 0.43 ($p < 0.05$ one-tailed).

Referring to the question which were the most realized art-of-living sub-constructs, Table 6.3 shows the most realized were *positive attitudes towards life*, *self-efficacy*, *openness*, *meaning*, *self-determined way of living* and *reflection*. The Spearman rank order correlations between art-of-living and realization resulted in 0.61 ($p < 0.05$ one-tailed).

A closer look to the sub-constructs listed in both ranked orders shows that for artists of living the ranked order of importance and realization of art-of-living were quite similar.

6.2.4.3 Qualitative Analysis

The mentions for attitudes and abilities that help to gain satisfaction in life were analyzed with a content analysis. In the first step, an open category system was developed on the basis of preliminary realizations which was then expanded and changed during the coding of the participants' answers. To ensure the accuracy of the coding, the answers were independently assigned to the final categories by two raters which afterwards discussed the discrepancies. The inter-rater-reliability was determined with Cohen's Kappa which was 0.918.

The 38 participants gave 213 answers to the question which were assigned to 23 categories. Figure 6.1 gives an overview of the answers.

The category with the most mentions was social competence, followed by openness, positive attitude and conscious living. Most of the mentioned aspects are contained in our concept of art-of-living we described in Chap. 1, although among the top ten categories were two which are not included in our concept, being confidence and courage. From our perspective, courage is contained in the catalog of Strength and Virtues, cf. Peterson and Seligman (2004) and we see no benefit in adding this aspect as a standalone sub-construct, because, as we discussed in Chap. 1, we tried to reduce the influence of moral values. The aspect of confidence could be helpful as a part of social contact. In sum, there is no great difference between our concept and what artists-of-living think about art-of-living.

The interview tried to find answers to questions such as what art-of-living means to the artists-of-living, which strategies they use to practice it and whether one is able to learn being an artist-of-living. In the following, explanatory extracts from answers to these questions will be presented.

One participant described art-of-living as "a piece of art that I am creating for myself. Every day and every moment, I am creating my own piece of art that is the life that I create. Like a sculptor, day after day beating off pieces of this great sculpture and then really creating a piece of art."

Another person stressed the importance of combining different aspects for art-of-living: "Living life, achieving something, but at the same time being able to enjoy things. There are many people who achieve something, but don't enjoy and

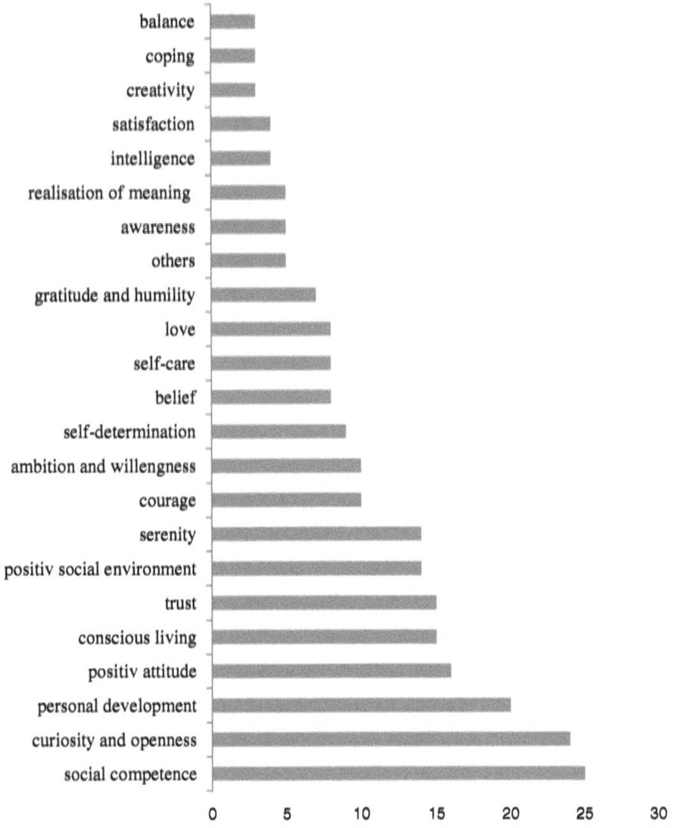

Fig. 6.1 Categories and their frequency for answers to the open questions

there are many people that enjoy a lot but don't achieve anything and to me it is the skill to combine both. And to do that with the greatest possible ease."

The participants did not only report their views of art-of-living, they also mentioned how it was reflected in their actions. One participant saw her vocation in providing support for others and therefore worked as a coach. Another mentioned the positive dealing with challenges and leaving room for topics such as spirituality despite a very tight schedule due to his autistic child.

It was also assumed that art-of-living is reflected by principles, values and attitudes in life that guide actions. These were very diverse and included serenity and humor as well as openness and honesty or living together with others and treating them appreciatively.

An important strategy was the constant reflection which means reflecting one's being, one's actions and one's goals and enables a person to lead a conscious life. The participants said that they were consciously looking for and creating a (social) environment that encourages and also demands practicing art-of-living and fits their own needs. Additionally, interaction served as inspiration for the reflection.

One participant said his strategy to get "out of the mental world and into the real life" was to learn "in the here and now" and practice to completely live in the moment focusing on small things. This can be achieved by daily, recurring activities such as eating very mindfully and consciously.

To another participant, gratefulness as the first and the last thought of the day is very important. Another strategy is "five minutes of silliness every day", which she learned from her mother and frequently passes on to others.

Some other statements were:

> May be that art-of-living can be seen as a process, a development. … To peel oneself like an onion, starting with what I lived as an adolescent, where I had around me a lot of unnatural layers. … With every year of my life to peel the layers and to approach art-of-living. Art-of-living can then be seen in the proper meaning of the word: that is my core, my fire, my inside.

> In this fast moving age with a seemingly endless number of possibilities seems the aptitude to concentrate on a few things to be important for a satisfying life.

> Art-of-living means not only to discuss but to act, to take hands on.

Others mentioned the relevance of openness and trying to *understand* what they do, to understand their friends and the function of the world.

There were also commentaries dealing with the questionnaire of art-of-living. Some persons criticize that it is more focused on an individual perspectives and that a transcendental view and "the big picture" is neglected.

6.2.5 Summary

Summarizing the nomination study, we could show that our procedure of nomination led to find a sample of artists-of-living. Analyses of their answers to the art-of-living questionnaire show that they differ from our normal sample with respect to the most but not all aspects of art-of-living. There were similarities between the ratings of importance/realization of the art-of-living sub-constructs and the results of the questionnaires. The answers regarding the open questions were quite interesting and gave an enriched picture of what artists-of-living understand by art-of-living. The main ideas of the artists-of-living fit with our concept, but these interviews also showed some topics which were neglected in our concept. One example for neglected themes was the process-perspective of art-of-living nicely expressed in an onion metaphor. Following this view art-of-living develops over time and its contours become more clearly. Because our questionnaire is conceptualized more as a trait instrument, the developmental aspect is difficult to grasp.

An example for a still imprecise conceptualization is the sub-construct of reflection, as, according to the questionnaire results, there is no difference between the amount artists-of-living reflect and normal people reflect, cf. Table 6.2, although artists-of-living rate reflection as important and claim they realize it in their life very often, cf. Table 6.3. We conclude, that the questionnaire does not measure the core part of reflection precisely enough.

Related to the concept of reflection is the idea of consciously living one's life, which implies to be mindful what is happing. Mindfulness is a concept related to art-of-living but still different because it signifies to observe what is happening nonjudgmentally. Living consciously also implies to focus on the "here and now" and to select and concentrate on what is important. Artists-of-living give the advice not only to observe but also to try to understand what is happening, to understand what one does oneself but also what other people do and how the world is functioning. Art-of-living should not be related only to the feeling of the individual but also to the relationships with friends and the society and the world as whole, therefore, one should not lose sight of the big picture. With respect to effort and trying to attain important goals one should not neglect aspects of joyfulness and savoring. In our model that means, to live single components of art-of-living will not be satisfying because one has to integrate different aspects of art-of-living. All in all, the metaphor of one artist-of-living fits our perspective: Life can be viewed as working on a piece of art where the artist is the actor working on himself and the piece of art at the same time.

6.3 Summary

Bernhard Schmitz

In the following, we will summarize the key points of every chapter in this book to give a summary on the book as a whole. Finally, we will give an outlook on questions still unanswered which provide ideas for further research.

6.3.1 Summing Up on the Introduction

In the introductory chapter we defined the criteria for our art-of-living model:

First, we understand art-of-living not as the outcome of leading a good life but as a predictor of well-being. Second, art-of-living should be conceptualized *not too general, not too fine-grained and not too moralistic*. Third, following Veenhoven (2003a, b), we argued that art-of-living can be performed *in many different ways* and each individual can find its own way. Fourth, we think that art-of-living includes *strategies as well as attitudes*. Fifth, we consider that *art-of-living can be learned* and especially certain aspects of it, meaning that *art-of-living can be realized by almost everyone*. Sixth, we wanted to show that *art-of-living can be measured with reliability and validity*. Seventh, we wanted to demonstrate *empirically that we can design interventions that can enhance art-of-living and happiness* for different groups and in different ways.

6.3.2 *Summary on the Questionnaire*

Pursuing the idea from Veenhovens (2003a, b) special issue in the Journal of Happiness Studies, we transferred the concept of art-of-living, which has a long tradition in philosophy, to psychological research. To achieve that, we conducted a study on the common understanding of art-of-living and merged the results with the philosophical background (particularly by Schmid 2004) to elaborate our concept of art-of-living with its corresponding subscales. That enabled us to develop a questionnaire as an empirical foundation for its measurement which was then evaluated on its susceptibility for social desirability, its internal consistency, its validation and its factorial structure.

We proved that the questionnaire is only minimally influenced by social desirability. Regarding internal consistency, the questionnaire showed satisfactory statistical properties like high overall internal consistency but also sufficient consistency for most of the subscales. As for validation purposes, there is a high correlation between the overall art-of-living scale and subjective well-being of $r = .69$, the multiple correlation of all the subscales was 0.78, and the R^2 value was 0.61, which shows that art-of-living and subjective well-being are connected but still distinct enough to be seen as different constructs. That also gives a hint that high art-of-living might lead to an increased feeling of well-being.

With respect to the factorial structure it was proved that it is beneficial to view art of living as an overall structure as well as to have a closer look on the subscales.

Investigating if people can be clustered to groups by the similarity of their profiles, latent class and cluster analyses showed that there are different subgroups, but that they are not defined through homogenous profiles, as the individual profiles were quite distinct, but rather through their different general level of art-of-living. This is in line with the view that there are many different ways to perform art-of-living (and also corresponding to Schmid 2004; Veenhoven 2003a, b).

Regarding the question whether art-of-living can be learned, we, along with Schmid and our sample, agree, that it is possible. Given that, the instrument we introduced could be used to assess the actual level of art-of-living for a person and thereby show possibilities for improvements. Using pre- and post-measurements the questionnaire could also be used to evaluate interventions that try to enhance art-of-living.

6.3.3 *Summary on the Validation*

After getting first results from the validation of the questionnaire with the construct of Subjective Well-Being (SWB) we wanted to further assess the validity of the instrument.

First, we tried to show that art-of-living is related to its goal, the attainment of well-being. We compared the relationships of the art-of-living-questionnaire with several questionnaires measuring happiness and well-being, namely the satisfaction with life scale (SWLS), the subjective happiness scale (SHS), the authentic happiness scale (AHI), psychological well-being (PWB) and eudaimonic well-being (EWB). The correlation was generally high (r = .62 for SHS and r = .69 for AHI. We also found a negative correlation to depression (Beck Depression Inventory, BDI), a construct which is often seen as the opposite of well-being or happiness.

Second, we investigated the relationship between art-of-living and flourishing which were highest to the Seligman's PERMA measure (r = .76).

Third, we studied the relationship between personality measured by the big 5 and art-of-living to find out whether art-of-living could be mainly determined by personality. Regarding personality the correlations between art-of-living and the big 5 were between 0.21 and −0.59. A multiple regression proved that well-being (SWLS) could partially be predicted by personality but art-of-living could add a significant and remarkable part for the prediction above personality (incremental validity).

Fourth, we studied the similarity between other ways aiming for leading a good life, being strength and virtues and orientations to happiness (OTH). The analyses of communalities between strength and virtues and art-of-living revealed all significant correlations and the highest correlations to transcendence and wisdom. With respect to OTH the art-of-living-strategies are significantly related to all orientations that means they provide strategies related to all the three orientations with a little higher relationship to engagement although no direct measure of engagement or flow is included in art-of-living.

Fifth, we analyzed the relationship between other important constructs of positive psychology resilience, sense of coherence, self-regulation and wisdom, which also yielded high correlations to art-of-living but it could be shown that art-of-living adds to each of these constructs to predict well-being.

We also showed that special subscales of art-of-living correlate with work-related variables like subjective occupational success or self-fulfillment in working life.

In addition to this content oriented validation we validated the self-report-questionnaire with other measures for art-of-living, namely peer estimation of art-of-living, which proved correlations of a magnitude comparable to that of similar measures, and a newly developed situational judgement test (SJT) of art-of-living, which showed encouraging results with respect to its consistency and its correlation with the self-report questionnaire.

In the end, we improved the first version of the questionnaire based on theoretical and empirical reasons. We changed items and added three scales and showed that all subscales had sufficient internal consistencies.

6.3.4 Summary of Process Analyses Based on Diary Data

Then we took steps for enabling the measurement of art-of-living in diary-studies.

We proposed a short art-of-living state-measure which would be beneficial for more frequent measures, e.g. for daily use in diary studies, and proved that this state measure shows high internal consistencies for the overall art-of-living measure as well as for the most of its subscales. In addition, by using the split-half-method (Schmitz and Skinner 1993), we proved that state art-of-living shows high stability-coefficients. The calculated validity coefficients between the art-of-living short version (as state measure) and art-of-living long version (as trait like measure) yielded high coefficients both for the overall measure as well as for most of the subscales.

That facilitates the use of the state art-of-living as a diary measure in process analyses. Primary process analyses showed that state art-of-living is connected to daily uplifts but not to daily hassles and that state art-of-living is highly related to positive and negative daily affect. It also turned out that state art-of-living and state well-being have a high synchronous relationship, although the relationships differed between individuals which we think is due to individual specificity. That supports the view that individual differences should more often be in the focus of evaluation instead of just generalizing results for which generalization might not be beneficial. The shorter art-of-living state version enables such research and opens up new possibilities for diary measures as well as individual and longitudinal studies in the context of art-of-living.

6.3.5 Summary of Intervention Studies

As yet, there is a need for studies on the effectiveness of art-of-living interventions. When focusing on the related theory of positive psychology, meta-analyses convincingly demonstrate that positive psychology interventions (ppi) are effective. But it is criticized that they are mainly presented as stand-alone interventions.

In our view it is fruitful to use interventions which holistically integrate a group of strategies. This is done within the concept of art-of-living which integrates sub-components with respect to the model and to the needs of the sample which is studied.

The studies we conducted all had different foci, used different interventions and were aiming at specific target groups, being university students, pupils and employees.

One study investigated special *combinations of training* contents, body related and cognitive interventions. Another study dealt with *the fit of person and kind of treatment assignment*, which proved that not self-selection of interventions but assignment based on deficits led to better results. Other studies tested a *work-based intervention* and the last a *web-based intervention*, which both were successful in changing important art-of-living aspects.

In the corresponding chapter, the applied interventions were described in greater detail than in many scientific publications as to encourage the application of the methods to other studies.

The data suggests that all conducted interventions were at least partially effective which supports the view that art-of-living can be learnt and proves that it is possible to enhance art-of-living components or overall art-of-living by short interventions for different target groups. Some follow-up tests indicated that the increase of art-of-living by the trainings was either stable or even further enhanced from the post- to the follow-up-testing.

6.3.6 Limitations

The concept of art-of-living is dealt with in philosophy since ancient times and was in recent years brought up again by W. Schmid and Veenhoven. We tried to transfer the concept of art-of-living from philosophy to psychology which was not easy because philosophical authors don't have the measurement of their constructs in mind when writing. To be able to measure it, we needed to simplify and reduce Schmids theories, which is a necessity looking at the fact that the elaboration of W. Schmid about the philosophy of art-of-living has more than 500 pages. That brings up the topic whether our approach of art-of-living fulfills the criterion of completeness. For example, whereas Schmid describes in detail ways of physical care like dancing, touching, fasting and breathing we only included one sub-construct for all these ways of physical care. Similarly he elaborates ways of care for oneself like self-attention, self-talk, self-friendship and self-management which we did not include in our concept, at least not under these labels. Therefore, the question of completeness is a difficult question, e.g. humor is definitely an important and successful strategy to achieve well-being, but from our perspective, humor could be subsumed under coping strategies or positive attitude towards life. But this kind of integration into the existing component structure cannot be unequivocally decided, there is room for interpretation which could lead to a discussion of the appropriate hierarchy of the constructs. In the introductory chapter we explained that we wanted to include constructs not too broad and not too narrow. One could solve this discussion by conceptualizing a hierarchy of constructs and sub-constructs as done for example in Eysenck and Eysenck (1976). For our purposes it seems to be too early to propose such a differentiated system.

Another criterion is that a model should be economical. Are all subcomponents really needed? This is also a difficult question, which could be answered using factor analyses and multiple regression to predict a desired criterion. But since different criteria could be applied, e.g. flourishing or eudaimonic well-being, that might lead to different results.

Another topic is the inclusion of negative conditions, e.g. Wong (2013) has proposed the dual system model which includes positive and negative conditions and outcomes, which has yet to be achieved in the context of art-of-living.

Also, in this book we looked mainly at well-being and flourishing as result of art-of-living, because that was our main goal and therefore, until now the *prediction* of art-of-living was not analyzed in detail. But it would be interesting to investigate whether art-of-living is dependent on certain conditions like income, education, family background and genetic influences etc.

In a similar direction one could ask for the cultural dependence of art-of-living. Whereas Peterson and Seligman (2004) tried to find culture independent strength and virtues, our approach for art-of-living seems, up until now, to be more oriented to Western values and traditions.

Furthermore, the evaluation of the *development of art-of-living over time* could be needed, but up to the actual status of the clarification of the construct it seems to be too early to study such phenomena.

6.3.7 Perspectives

We do not assume that our concept will be the final answer to the question how art-of-living can be conceptualized and measured. We rather believe that it is a good starting point in supporting the development of the psychological study of art-of-living on an empirical basis.

We presented a lot of evidence that art-of-living is a construct which can be measured reliably and shows systematic relationships within a nomological network of related constructs. Our questionnaire seems to be useful, but it may be too long to be suited for easy and economic measurement of art-of-living. The interventions for students in school, for university students and employees seem to be effective although studies with greater samples and other combinations of sub-constructs might be necessary.

Future studies might further sharpen the contours of the concept and its measurement and ways to enhancement. Art-of-living could be seen as a good way for living a good life but not the only one.

References

Atteslander, P. (2010). *Methoden qualitativer Sozialforschung*.

Baltes, P. B., & Staudinger, U. M. (2000). Wisdom: A metaheuristic (pragmatic) to orchestrate mind and virtue toward excellence. *American Psychologist, 55*, 122–136.

Baltes, P., Staudinger, U. M., Maercker, A., & Smith, J. (1995). People nominated as wise: A comparative study of wisdom-related knowledge. *Psychology and Aging*, 155–166.

Clapton, E., & Sykes, C. S. (2007). *Eric Clapton: The autobiography*. New York: Random House.

Dalai Lama. (2011). *My spiritual autobiography*. Rider.

Eysenck, H. J., & Eysenck, S. B. G. (1976). *Psychoticism as a dimension of personality*. London: Hodder and Stoughton Educational.

Häder, M. (Ed.). (2002). *Delphi-Befragungen. Ein Arbeitsbuch*. Wiesbaden: Westdt. Verlag.

Mandela, N. R. (1995). *Long walk to freedom*. Back Bay Books

Niemiec, R. M., & Wedding, D. (2008). Positive psychology at the movies. *Using films to build virtues and character strenghts*. Hogrefe.

Niemiec, R. M., Wedding, D., & Monfries, M. (2014). Positive Psychology at the movies 2: *Using films to build character strengths and well-being*.

Pavarotti, L., & Wright, W. (1998). *Pavarotti: My world*. Arrow Books.

Peterson, C., & Seligman, M. E. (2004). *Character strengths and virtues: A handbook and classification*. Oxford: Oxford University Press.

Schmid, W. (2004). *To be friends with ourselves—About the art of living with oneself*. Suhrkamp Publishers.

Schmitz, B., & Skinner, E. (1993). Perceived control, effort, and academic performance: Interindividual, intraindividual, and multivariate time-series analyses. *Journal of Personality and Social Psychology, 64*(6), 1010.

Schnell, H., & Hill, P. B. (2013). Esser (2011): Methoden der empirischen Sozialforschung. *Auflage, München, 201*(1)

Thoreau, H. D. (2014). *Walden*. Black & White Classics.

Veenhoven, R. (2003a). Arts-of-living. *Journal of Happiness Studies* (4), 373–384.

Veenhoven, R. (2003b). Notions of art-of-living. *Journal of Happiness Studies, 4*(4), 345–349.

Wong, P. T. (Ed.). (2013). *The human quest for meaning: Theories, research, and applications*. London: Routledge.

MIX
Papier aus verantwortungsvollen Quellen
Paper from responsible sources
FSC® C105338

If you have any concerns about our products,
you can contact us on
ProductSafety@springernature.com

In case Publisher is established outside the EU,
the EU authorized representative is:
Springer Nature Customer Service Center GmbH
Europaplatz 3, 69115 Heidelberg, Germany

Printed by Libri Plureos GmbH
in Hamburg, Germany